KETOGENIC DIET ON A BUDGET

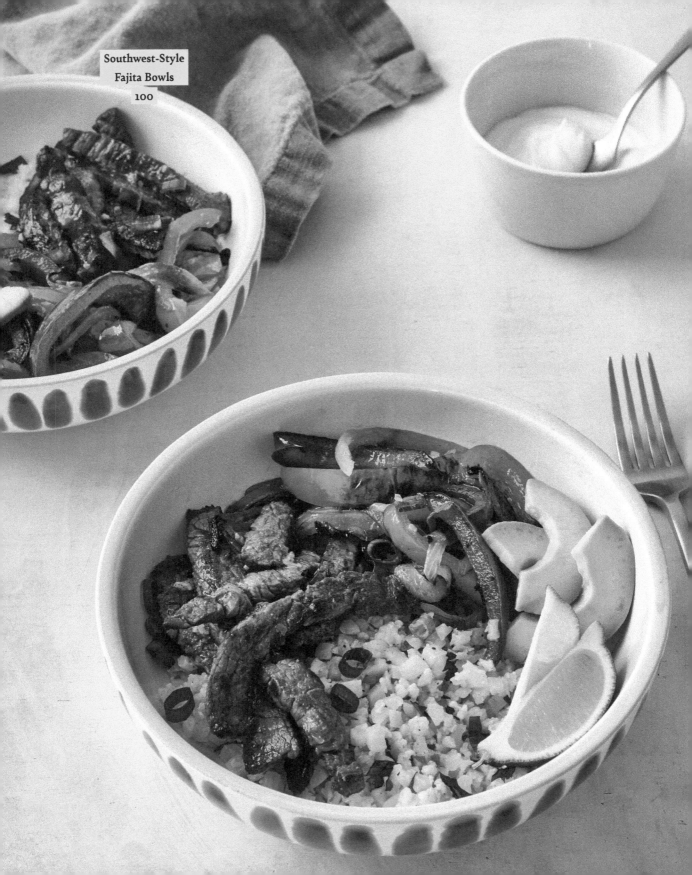

Ketogenic Diet
ON A BUDGET

Shop Smarter, Batch Cook, and Eat Better

Wes Shoemaker

Photography by Kate Sears

ROCKRIDGE PRESS

To Joshua, for being my taste tester for the last 25 years—and my biggest cheerleader when I couldn't cheer for myself.

For general information on our other products and services or to obtain technical support, please contact our Customer Care Department within the United States at (866) 744-2665, or outside the United States at (510) 253-0500.

Rockridge Press publishes its books in a variety of electronic and print formats. Some content that appears in print may not be available in electronic books, and vice versa.

Interior and Cover Designer: Rachel Haeseker
Art Producer: Meg Baggott
Editor: Marjorie DeWitt
Production Editor: Andrew Yackira

Photography © 2021 Kate Sears. Food styling by Lori Powell.
Author photo courtesy of Irvin Rivera / graphicsmetropolis.

ISBN: Print 978-1-64611-206-7
eBook 978-1-64611-207-4

R0

Contents

Introduction
vii

CHAPTER 1
Going Keto without
Going Broke
1

CHAPTER 2
Breakfast
13

CHAPTER 3
Soups and
Salads
27

CHAPTER 4
Vegetables
45

CHAPTER 5
Poultry and
Seafood
61

CHAPTER 6
Meat
81

CHAPTER 7
Sweets and
Treats
103

CHAPTER 8
Keto Staples
119

Measurement Conversions
135

Index
136

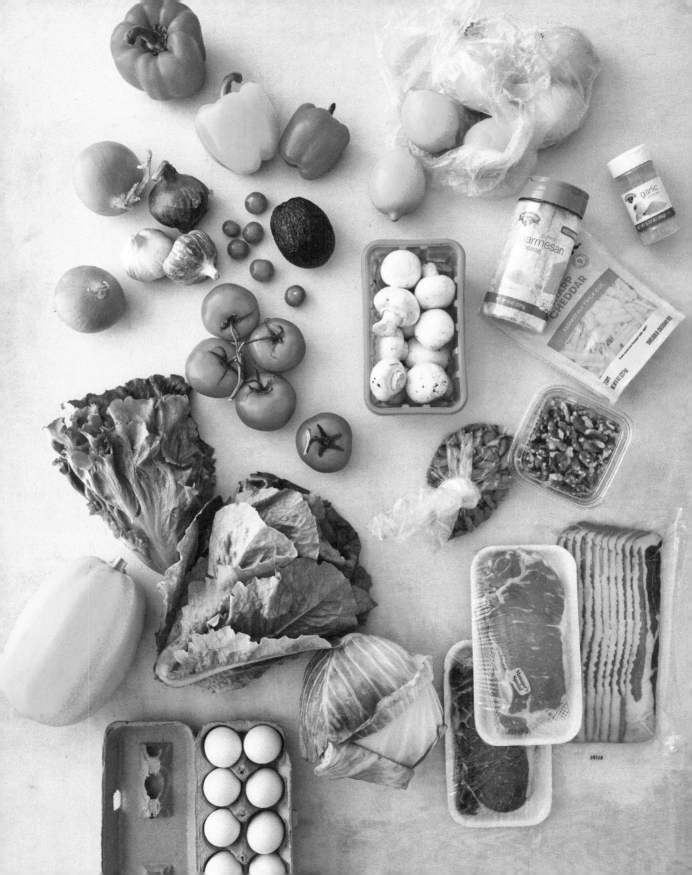

Introduction

Several years ago, when I started my keto journey, I created a YouTube channel called *Highfalutin' Low Carb* as a way to share recipes and ideas. It quickly grew into an amazing community of keto and low-carb eaters helping each other stay committed. My most popular videos are "Recipe Battles," where I make and test several keto recipes for a particular food (keto bread or keto cinnamon rolls, for instance) and determine a winner. With almost half a million social media followers at the time of this publication, one recurring comment I receive is a variation of: *"Thank you for saving me time and money. I waste so many expensive ingredients making recipes that turn out poorly, so now I always check your channel first."*

With that in mind, I set out to create a cookbook full of deliciously nourishing keto recipes that won't break the bank. Many keto recipes in cookbooks and online are full of unusual or expensive ingredients that might be rarely used or don't give the results promised. There's no need to waste time and money to eat a healthy ketogenic diet. The recipes in this book are delicious, easy, and affordable. This book will help you expand your palate and gain a solid understanding of the keto diet while using readily available ingredients you can find at any grocery store. Eating a ketogenic diet doesn't mean we have to spend a fortune; we just need to be smart about selecting recipes and ingredients.

Daily, I hear from followers who have struggled with starting, or sticking to, a keto diet. I have often felt that way myself, but I also know the tremendous rewards a ketogenic diet can bring. By sharing some tips and strategies, I'm hopeful that I can make this an easy and affordable journey for you and your family. Together we will meet our dietary goals—whether that's weight loss, improved health, decreased inflammation, or all of the above. I'm glad you're here. Let's get started!

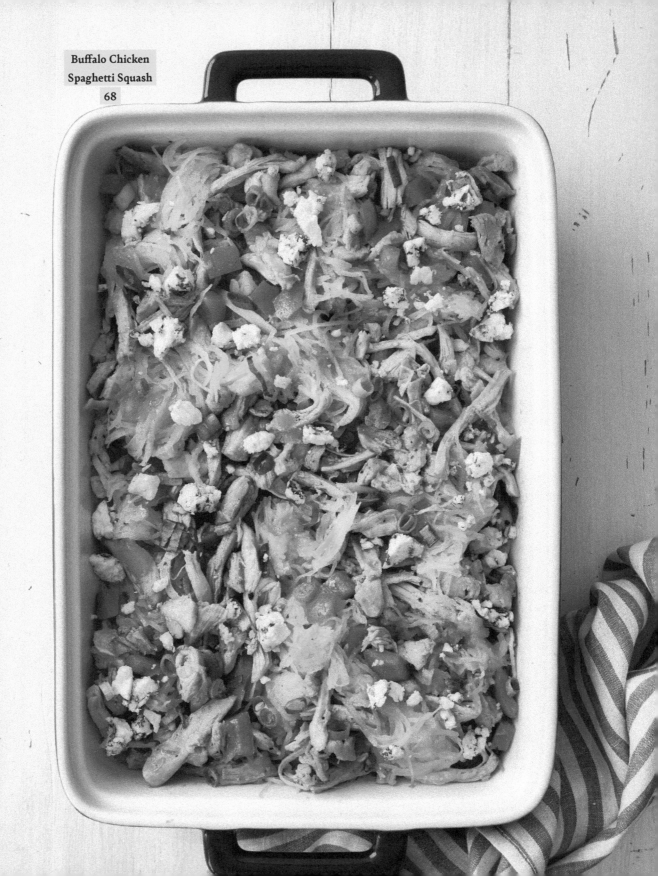

CHAPTER 1

Going Keto without Going Broke

Whether you're new to the ketogenic diet or a seasoned keto eater searching for budget-friendly recipes, the basics in this chapter will set you on a course for nutritional success. There are a few key elements to the keto way of eating that are essential to understand and remember if you want to feel great while losing weight or keeping the pounds off. Let's explore these points a bit further.

Why the Keto Diet Works (Even on a Budget)

By learning the ketogenic diet's core principles, you'll better understand how to manipulate the daily macronutrients ("macros") that you eat. Everything humans eat can be calculated into three main categories of macros: carbohydrates, proteins, and fats. Understanding how your body responds to each is the key to successfully navigating the ketogenic diet.

The Standard American Diet (typical Western diet) generally consists of around 2,000 calories a day, with 50 percent of those calories coming from carbohydrates, 15 percent from proteins, and 35 percent from fats. Scientists and nutritionists have told us for years that to lose weight and eat healthy, most of our diet should consist of complex carbohydrates and minimal fat. Modern scientific studies (and the increasing waist sizes and metabolic diseases rampant in Western society) now show us that, as a population, we've been eating too many carbs.

The ketogenic diet turns that old way of thinking about healthy nutrition on its head. Instead of getting most of your calories from carbs—which your body breaks down into glucose that you use as fuel—a keto diet uses fat as the main source of energy. In a typical ketogenic diet, the macros should be around 70 percent fat, 20 percent protein, and a mere 5 percent carbs. This means that instead of burning glucose for energy, you will now be burning fat through the process of ketosis. When you restrict your carb intake this much (and in turn your glucose), your body manufactures ketones to use as an energy source. When it does, you enter a healthy state of nutritional ketosis, which has countless benefits you've probably already heard about and are here to experience yourself: weight loss; mental clarity; management of inflammation, insulin sensitivity, and autoimmune disorders; and many others we will explore.

The goal of a ketogenic diet is to keep the body in a healthy state of ketosis at all times. Many people use expensive cuts of meats, exotic-sounding fats and oils, and costly supplements to maintain their ketogenic way of eating. But it doesn't have to be an expensive venture. You can follow a keto diet using simple ingredients you can find at any grocery store. Eggs, nuts, and affordable cuts of meat make great protein sources. Good-quality olive oil, butter, and avocados make fantastic healthy fat sources, and leafy greens and cruciferous vegetables should provide the few carbs you'll be eating each day. It just takes a little forethought and planning to make the keto diet sustainable, delicious, and affordable.

How Can I Tell If I'm in Ketosis?

Once you're following the guidelines of a keto diet, your body will give you some clues as you enter ketosis. One of the most commonly experienced is the often-dreaded "keto flu." This usually happens two to three days after restricting your carb intake. As your body adjusts to its new fuel source and depletes its glycogen stores, you'll likely feel tired, irritable, nauseated, have difficulty concentrating, and experience sugar cravings. This is normal and will go away within a week or less. Don't give up. It's a sure sign that your body is becoming fat adapted, and better days are on the horizon.

Another common sign of ketosis is a noticeable metallic taste in your mouth, which often comes with a bit of bad breath. (Don't worry, it's usually temporary.) As the body burns ketones, it can cause a fruity acetone odor to be expelled from the lungs. I've heard it described as a "copper penny" taste. Just keep some sugar-free breath mints or gum with you if it bothers you.

To find out exactly how deep you are in ketosis, there are tests available to measure ketones, including blood droplet monitors and electronic breathalyzers. They can be costly, and unless you're of a curious nature, neither are necessary. I advise against urine-strip tests. These are only useful right at the beginning of entering ketosis, as your body is "tossing away" ketones in your urine. Within a short time, your body will start to burn those ketones as fuel instead of getting rid of them, and the test strips become useless. My advice is simply to be aware of the most common signs of ketosis and trust that when you're experiencing them, you're on the right path.

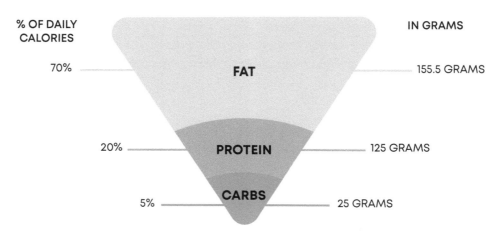

2,000-CALORIE DAILY KETOGENIC DIET

% OF DAILY CALORIES

IN GRAMS

70% — FAT — 155.5 GRAMS

20% — PROTEIN — 125 GRAMS

5% — CARBS — 25 GRAMS

A Thrifty Guide to the Keto Ratio

Maintaining ketosis is all about keeping a ratio of macronutrients in your diet. Fats, carbohydrates, and proteins each provide a specific amount of energy (calories) per gram. Carbohydrates and proteins both have 4 calories per gram, whereas fats have a whopping 9 calories per gram. Knowing this, you can see how fat is higher in energy than the other macros. This is why most of your daily calories should come from healthy fats. It can be difficult to overcome the "high-carb, low-fat" mantra we were told for so long, but trust that you can make the switch and live a healthier lifestyle while still eating delicious food. Gone are the days of the blood sugar roller coaster of crashes and cravings that many of us know all too well.

Everyone's individual caloric requirements will vary based on body weight, goal weight, activity level, and general metabolism. So, it's important to know how many calories you need to eat each day to achieve your goals. I usually tell people to go to any internet search engine and type in "keto calculator" and select one to try. There are many great free options; just make sure to select one that is geared toward a ketogenic diet and that isn't pushing a product or service. After entering some basic information like height, weight, goal weight, and activity level, the online calculator will provide a rough guideline of the calories and macros you should eat each day.

Many people like (or need) to track their macros, especially when just starting a keto journey. If you track what you eat each day and tally the macros for each item, you can ensure that you remain in ketosis. It's certainly possible to calculate it by hand, but it's even easier to use a smartphone app such as Carb Manager or Lose It. These allow you to select foods from a large database and keep a running calculation of your macros and calories, showing you how closely you're adhering to your specific goals.

Let's discuss the three macro categories, how much of your diet should come from each category, and some examples of healthy, affordable options.

FAT

As mentioned earlier, you'll need to get about 70 percent of your calories each day from fat. Again, that might sound counterintuitive to everything you've heard in the past, but this is the basis of a healthy ketogenic diet. Because fat will be your main calorie source, it's important to consume healthy options, such as extra-virgin olive oil, butter (grass fed, if possible), heavy cream, and avocados. This category might be where you splurge on the healthiest available options. Steer clear of vegetable oil, canola oil, and corn oil; these are unhealthy fats and should be avoided.

PROTEINS

Proteins will make up around 20 percent of your diet. It's easy to go overboard with protein, so be mindful of serving sizes. Good budget-friendly options include eggs, chicken (particularly legs and thighs, which are fattier cuts), bacon, and ground beef.

CARBOHYDRATES

Carbohydrates will make up a scant 5 percent of your diet. Most people try to stay around 20 grams or less per day to maintain ketosis. Cutting out sugar, bread, pasta, rice, and potatoes will naturally reduce your carb intake a great deal. The few carbs allowed on a keto diet should come from vegetables and certain low-sugar fruits, so you get the vitamins and nutrients you need. Broccoli, asparagus, cauliflower, and small servings of berries (e.g., blueberries and raspberries) are all good options.

Keto Splurge/Steal

There are certain items that keto eaters tend to splurge on, but many of them have budget-friendly options if you know where to look.

Duck fat and beef tallow: Fancy fats are all the rage in keto cooking because they provide depth of flavor to all sorts of dishes, but you can create amazing flavor using rendered bacon fat, which is much cheaper and can be used in almost any recipe.

Keto sweeteners: Brand-name keto-friendly sweeteners such as Swerve or Lakanto can be pricey when purchased at your local grocery store. I often buy generic erythritol and stevia from online retailers such as Amazon and Netrition.com at a fraction of the cost.

Nuts: Almonds and macadamia nuts are keto friendly but pricey. Instead of prepackaged nuts, head over to the bulk section of your local supermarket where you can purchase any amount you want at a much lower cost.

Seafood: Fresh seafood is delicious but also expensive. Get your seafood fix without breaking the bank by using canned lump crabmeat or shrimp.

Steak: Got a craving for steak? Don't go immediately for a rib eye or filet. Look for cheaper options, such as a roast or hanger steak. If you can't shake that rib-eye desire, buy them in bulk at big-box stores, such as Costco or Sam's Club, and portion them for freezing. The initial purchase will cost more, but the price per pound will be less than half that of a typical grocery store.

Keto Shopping on a Budget

One of the best budget-saving tips I can offer is to be strategic about shopping. Wandering through grocery aisles trying to decide what's for dinner is the surest way to waste money. A better method is to plan what meals you'll make for the week (or perhaps a few weeks) and create a shopping list. This provides two benefits: You can check your pantry and freezer to see if you already have any of the items you need to make the recipes, and it allows you to enter the grocery store with a plan. Both of these prevent impulse buys, which are the nemesis of sticking to a budget. If your pantry is already stocked with some basic keto staples, you can buy ingredients for a whole week's worth of keto meals for less than $60. In fact, a full weeklong meal plan that included the Sausage and Cheese Frittata (page 14), Keto Beef Chili (page 35), Keto Lasagna (page 94), and Lemon Poppy Seed Muffins (page 104) cost me $55.

BIG-BOX STORES

Discount stores such as Costco, Sam's Club, and BJ's Wholesale usually require a membership fee to join, but the savings you accrue over the year can be substantial because they sell items in bulk. If you have the storage space, you can save a tremendous amount of money purchasing large quantities of meat, nuts, healthy fats, and frozen vegetables. Bring them home, divide them into the portion sizes you need, and store or freeze them. You can essentially "shop" from your own freezer and pantry each week.

CANS, BAGS, AND BINS

Almost every grocery store has a bin section where you can purchase any amount of an item, weigh it, and pay by the pound. These options are usually much cheaper than their prepackaged counterparts. This is a great technique for saving money on nuts, seeds, and other dry goods. Canned foods are also a fantastic way to lower the bill. Canned tuna, chicken, salmon, lump crabmeat, and salad shrimp are pantry staples I always have on hand.

SALES

This idea may seem like simple common sense, but be sure to check store sales for bargains, not only for manufacturer discounts but also in-store sales on meat and vegetables. Many stores feature a particular day of the week that offers "buy one get one" sales on meat that make it smart to stock up. Also, check the butcher areas for expensive cuts nearing expiration. They're perfectly safe to eat, but the store needs to get rid of them quickly, usually at deep discounts. Instead of purchasing a warm rotisserie chicken, head over to the cold section of the deli where you can pick up one left over from the day before at half the price. It's perfect for dividing up thighs for dinner tonight and breasts to make chicken salad for tomorrow's lunch.

STORE BRANDS

Generic store brands are often as good as or better than name brands. For example, one of the hardest products to find is marinara sauce without added sugar. Most brands are full of added carbs and sugar, but one popular keto option is Rao's Homemade Marinara Sauce. It's delicious and, used sparingly, is one of the lowest-carb pasta sauces. But it can be extremely pricey. A nice alternative is the Great Value brand sauce from Walmart, which is lower in carb count, just as tasty, and much less expensive. The same applies to good-quality oils and fats. Never be afraid to search your store's own brand for alternatives to more expensive brand names. (They're sometimes even manufactured by the same companies!)

WHAT'S IN SEASON?

Seasonality in the produce section creates a tremendous variability in cost. Shipping in out-of-season vegetables from hundreds or thousands of miles away is costly—not only in terms of price but also nutrients. Out-of-season produce is picked days or weeks before it's ripe and then ripened on the trip to your supermarket. It's often cheaper and healthier to purchase those vegetables frozen because they were picked at their peak ripeness and flash frozen. Look for produce that is in season in your area and lean toward those items. Zucchini and squash are warm-weather vegetables, whereas broccoli and cauliflower are cool-weather vegetables. Shop by season for savings.

Batch-and-Freeze Cooking 101

Besides smart shopping, another great way to save time and money is batch cooking. Instead of cooking each meal separately, consider designating one day of the week to cook a large batch of several recipes that can be portioned and then refrigerated or frozen. It makes busy weeknight meals easy because you can simply reheat and serve.

You'll need some reusable containers for freezing. For larger portions, take them out of the freezer and place in the refrigerator to thaw overnight. For single items, like keto empanadas or cookies, for instance, place them individually on a sheet pan in the freezer. When frozen, transfer them to a zip-top bag and store in the freezer. This makes it easy to remove individual servings for reheating.

Batch cooking isn't just for recipes; it can also be for individual ingredients. For instance, cook up a few pounds of ground beef using simple seasonings like salt and pepper. Then you can use it multiple times in a week. For example, when reheating, you can add Southwest seasonings for taco salads one night and Italian seasonings for zucchini noodle Bolognese another night.

Batch cooking is a fantastic way to save time and money, reduce waste, and keep you on track on those nights when you don't feel like cooking and you start eyeing the takeout menus. Don't think of batch cooking as a chore. Get together with a friend or family member who's also eating keto, and each make a couple of your favorite recipes. Divide them up and swap so you have a variety of meals to enjoy.

Kitchen Staples

There are a few key foods that are always good to have in your keto kitchen. Here are a few items I regularly have on hand.

Canned goods
- Chicken breast
- Lump crabmeat
- Pink salmon
- Salad shrimp
- Tuna in olive oil

Fresh Dairy
- Butter
- Cream cheese
- Eggs
- Heavy cream
- Shredded cheeses (mozzarella and cheddar)

Fresh Produce
- Asparagus
- Avocados
- Bell peppers
- Cauliflower
- Cucumbers
- Scallions
- Zucchini

Frozen Produce

- Broccoli
- Brussels sprouts
- Cauliflower
- Mixed berries

Frozen Meats

- Bacon, uncured
- Beef, ground (80/20)
- Chicken thighs
- Shrimp, raw, peeled and deveined

Nuts

- Almonds, raw
- Macadamia nuts

Pantry Staples

- Almond and/or coconut flour
- Coconut oil
- Mayonnaise
- Olive oil
- Pork rinds (for breading)

Essential Kitchen Equipment

You don't need any special equipment to make the recipes in this book. There are a few items that you will likely need, and I've listed them here. If there's an item you don't have (or something you'd like to splurge on, e.g., a blender or food processor), look for it at thrift stores and yard sales. You can get gently used kitchen equipment for a fraction of the price of new.

9-by-13-inch casserole dish: You'll use this often for oven-baked casseroles and roasting vegetables and meats.

Measuring cups and spoons: A set of dry measuring cups and one liquid measuring cup are ideal.

Saucepans: A smaller 2-quart and larger 4-quart saucepan will ensure that you can steam vegetables and make sauces.

Sheet pan: This is essential for roasting meats and vegetables as well as baking keto desserts.

Skillet: Whether nonstick, stainless steel, or cast iron, a skillet is essential for searing meats.

Stockpot with lid: You'll use this often for soups, stews, and batch cooking large recipes.

Utensils: These are essential: spatula, large mixing spoon, vegetable peeler (for zucchini noodles), large chef's knife, small paring knife, cutting board, parchment paper, and box grater (for ricing cauliflower and grating cheese).

And here are a few items that are nice to have but not essential: Blender or food processor, hand mixer, rolling pin, steamer basket insert, muffin tin, loaf pan, and electric multicooker.

The Recipes in This Book

I've included recipes that taste great and will keep you satiated. But more importantly, these recipes are designed to maintain your state of ketosis and to be made with inexpensive ingredients that can be found in any grocery store. The price per serving for many of these recipes is on average $3 or less.

The recipes here are a mix of stand-alone meals, e.g., Chicken Divan Casserole (page 66), and mix-and-match meals you can put together as you see fit, such as Pan-Seared Hanger Steak with Easy Herb Cream Sauce (page 83) and Roasted Green Bean Almandine with Blistered Tomatoes (page 48). I also wanted to give you the most bang for your buck when it comes to cooking time and expense. Most of the recipes in this book will feed six to eight people, so they are great for a big crowd, a hungry family, or for portioning out to freeze or refrigerate and reheat later. Some of the recipes include instructions for using an electric pressure multicooker, but I also include alternative cooking methods if you don't have a multicooker.

I've also provided some tips and tricks along the way for working with ingredients and tools and helping with meal planning and batch cooking. When possible, I've included alternative ingredients to convert a recipe to vegetarian or dairy- or nut-free. You'll also find a **Super Saver** label that I've applied to recipes that are under $2 per serving. Lastly, each recipe includes full macro calculations and ratios to help you plan your meals and maintain ketosis.

I hope you enjoy these delicious meals as much as I do!

SUPER SAVER

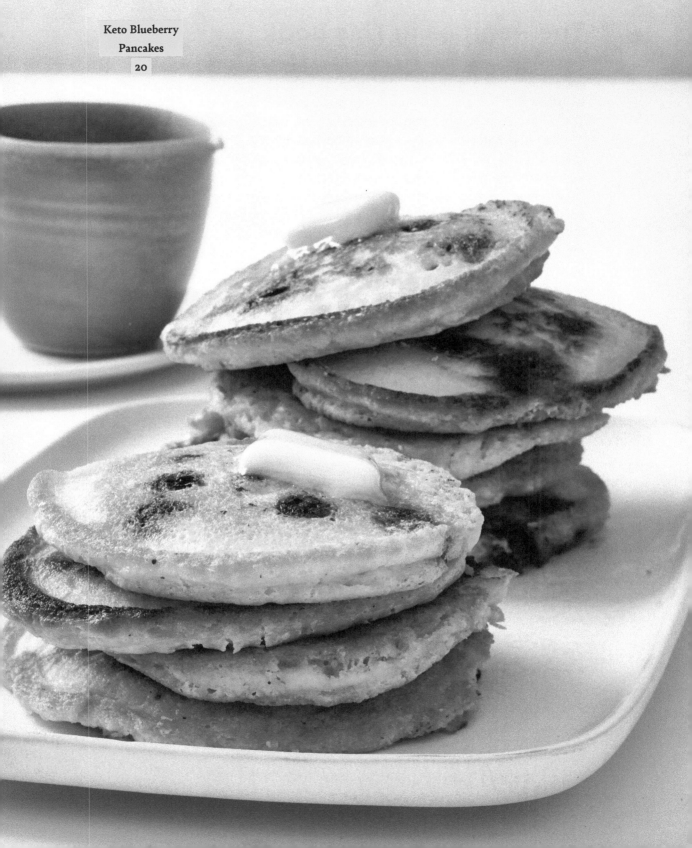

CHAPTER 2

Breakfast

Sausage and Cheese Frittata 14

Bacon Broccoli Crustless Quiche Cups 15

Breakfast Burrito Bowl 17

Overnight Chocolate Chia Pudding 18

Salmon and Egg Scramble 19

Keto Blueberry Pancakes 20

Ham and Cheese Egg Cups 21

Classic Diner Hash Browns 23

Baked Egg Avocado Boats 24

Cheesy Sausage and Cabbage Hash 25

Sausage and Cheese Frittata

Serves 8
Prep time: 10 minutes

Cook time: 35 minutes
Total time: 45 minutes

This oven-baked frittata reminds me of those universally loved breakfast casseroles; it's easy to make for a large crowd and also perfect for portioning for several weekday breakfasts. With sausage, butter, and cream, it satisfies the fat macros as well as the taste buds. For an even fluffier, creamier texture, you can use a blender instead of a whisk to combine the liquid ingredients.

4 tablespoons butter, melted, plus more for greasing pan
10 eggs
¾ cup heavy cream
½ teaspoon garlic powder
½ teaspoon onion powder
½ teaspoon paprika

½ teaspoon salt
½ teaspoon freshly ground black pepper
1 or 2 dashes favorite hot sauce (optional)
½ cup shredded cheddar cheese
1 cup cooked ground breakfast sausage
½ cup diced scallion
½ cup diced red bell pepper

1. Preheat the oven to 350°F.

2. Grease a 9-by-13-inch glass casserole dish with butter or cooking spray.

3. In a large bowl, whisk together the eggs, cream, butter, garlic powder, onion powder, paprika, salt, pepper, hot sauce (if using), and cheddar until well combined. Pour into the prepared casserole dish.

4. Evenly distribute the sausage, scallion, and bell pepper into the egg mixture.

5. Place on the center rack of the oven and bake for 35 minutes or until the frittata is cooked through and the top is very lightly browned.

6. Allow to rest for 5 minutes and serve.

INGREDIENT TIP: Instead of cooking the sausage from raw, I often use frozen, precooked breakfast sausage patties. It costs about the same, but it's more convenient for smaller amounts. Just defrost 3 or 4 patties in the microwave and dice into small pieces.

Per serving: Calories: 284; Total Fat: 25g; Total Carbs: 2g; Fiber: 0g; Net Carbs: 2g; Protein: 12g
Macronutrients: Fat: 78%; Protein: 19%; Carbs: 3%

Bacon Broccoli Crustless Quiche Cups

Makes 12
Prep time: 10 minutes

Cook time: 20 minutes
Total time: 30 minutes

These delicious little quiche cups are fantastic for batch cooking for a week of quick breakfasts. Simply reheat in the microwave at 50 percent power for 30 to 40 seconds. This recipe also serves well as a base for other ingredients. You can easily swap out the broccoli and bacon for other fillings. Try diced mushroom and deli ham, or diced bell pepper and chopped baby spinach for a vegetarian alternative.

Nonstick cooking spray
1 cup chopped fresh broccoli
1 cup shredded cheddar or pepper
    Jack cheese
½ cup chopped cooked bacon

8 eggs
½ cup heavy cream
½ teaspoon onion powder
½ teaspoon salt
½ teaspoon freshly ground black pepper

1. Preheat the oven to 350°F.

2. Thoroughly coat the cups of a 12-cup muffin tin with cooking spray.

3. Evenly divide the broccoli, cheese, and bacon between the muffin cups.

4. In a large bowl, whisk together the eggs, cream, onion powder, salt, and pepper until well combined. Pour the egg mixture into the muffin cups, distributing it evenly.

5. Bake for 18 minutes or until set. Allow to rest, then carefully remove each cup with a fork and large spoon that will fit around it.

BATCH-COOKING TIP: If you like your breakfast to go, place paper muffin liners in the tin before spraying with cooking spray. This makes them finger friendly for on-the-go eating. Store leftover quiche cups in a zip-top bag in the freezer for up to 3 months.

Per serving: Calories: 143; Total Fat: 12g; Total Carbs: 1g; Fiber: 0g; Net Carbs: 1g; Protein: 8g
Macronutrients: Fat: 74%; Protein: 24%; Carbs: 2%

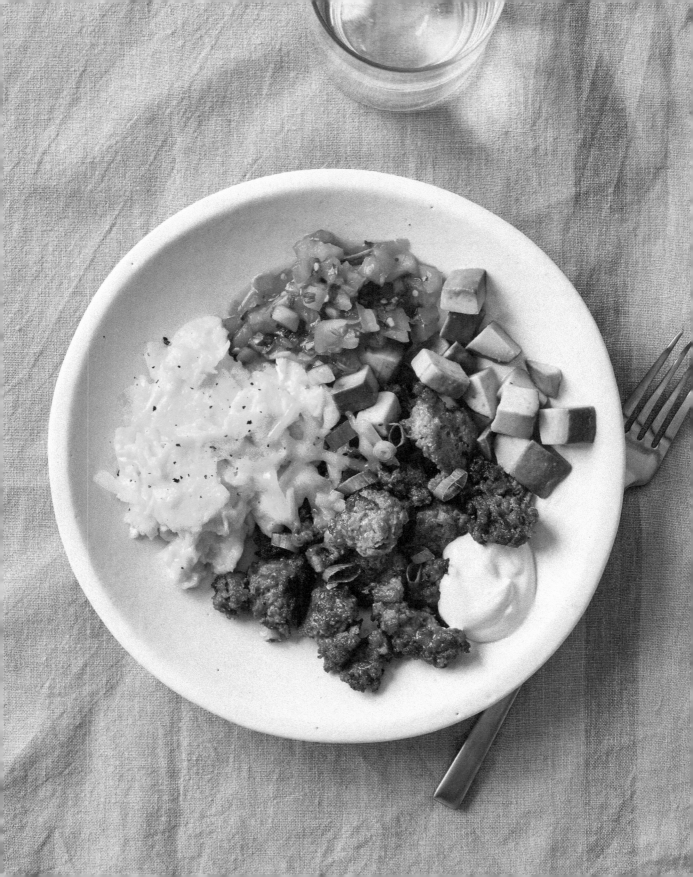

Breakfast Burrito Bowl

Serves 6
Prep time: 5 minutes

Cook time: 15 minutes
Total time: 20 minutes

Burrito bowls are a great way to get the flavors and textures of a breakfast burrito without the carbs of a tortilla. I love the ease of this dish and how it provides a little more interest than just scrambled eggs and sausage. Be sure to select a salsa with no added sugar and use it sparingly for flavor. Fresh salsas in the produce aisle are often better alternatives than jarred salsa for this reason, but they won't last as long in the refrigerator.

1 pound breakfast sausage
8 eggs, beaten
Salt
Freshly ground black pepper
1 cup shredded cheddar cheese

1 avocado, diced
½ cup salsa
½ cup sour cream
2 or 3 scallions, sliced

1. In a large skillet over medium heat, cook the breakfast sausage, breaking it up into small pieces, until browned. Remove from the skillet and divide between 6 bowls.

2. In a medium bowl, beat the eggs and lightly season with salt and pepper.

3. Pour off all but about 1 tablespoon of fat from the skillet.

4. Add the beaten eggs to the skillet and cook over medium heat, stirring regularly to scramble. Divide the eggs between the 6 bowls.

5. Top each bowl with the cheese, avocado, salsa, sour cream, and scallions.

Per serving: Calories: 455; Total Fat: 35g; Total Carbs: 8g; Fiber: 3g; Net Carbs: 5g; Protein: 26g
Macronutrients: Fat: 70%; Protein: 23%; Carbs: 7%

Overnight Chocolate Chia Pudding

Makes 6   **Prep time:** 5 minutes, plus overnight to chill

Chia seeds are tiny nutritional superstars packed with vitamins, minerals, antioxidants, protein, and fiber. If you enjoy the texture of traditional tapioca or rice pudding, there's a good chance you'll love this amazing keto alternative. It's about as simple as it gets—just mix, refrigerate, and wait. The carbohydrate count of chia seeds initially seems high, but it's almost all fiber, which is subtracted from total carb count to get net carb count. (Net carbs are what most people on a keto diet calculate.) Store these puddings covered in the refrigerator for up to five days.

4½ cups unsweetened almond milk
9 tablespoons chia seeds
6 tablespoons unsweetened cocoa powder

1 sweetener of choice:
- 3 packets Splenda, or
- 10 to 12 drops liquid stevia, or
- 3 tablespoons sugar-free Torani syrup, or
- 3 tablespoons powdered erythritol blend

1. In a bowl, mix together all the ingredients until well combined.

2. Divide the mixture evenly between 6 (8-ounce or larger) glasses or canning jars.

3. Cover and refrigerate overnight.

4. The next morning, stir and serve.

Per serving: Calories: 169; Total Fat: 9g; Total Carbs: 18g; Fiber: 9g; Net Carbs: 9g; Protein: 4g; Erythritol: 6g
Macronutrients: Fat: 48%; Protein: 10%; Carbs: 42%

Salmon and Egg Scramble

Serves 6

Prep time: 5 minutes

Cook time: 10 minutes

Total time: 15 minutes

I was introduced to this delicious combination years ago by a dear friend, and I admit to having been skeptical. Fish and scrambled eggs didn't sound like a natural combo, but this dish has become a brunch staple in our house. Creamy, buttery scrambled eggs dotted with pink flakes of fresh salmon are as beautiful as they are delicious. Fresh salmon fillets might be a splurge, but I can often find single, small fillets, like the one needed here, for around $5 in the seafood section of my local grocery store.

8 eggs

2 tablespoons heavy cream

¼ teaspoon salt

¼ teaspoon freshly ground black pepper

4 tablespoons butter

1 (6-ounce) salmon fillet, skinned and diced into small slivers

1. In a bowl, thoroughly whisk together the eggs, cream, salt, and pepper.

2. In a large nonstick skillet over medium heat, melt the butter.

3. Add the eggs and salmon to the pan and cook over medium heat for 6 to 8 minutes or until the eggs are softly scrambled and the salmon pieces are cooked. Stir constantly to create creamy scrambled eggs.

SUBSTITUTION TIP: This dish is truly best with fresh salmon. But if it's too pricey, look for prepackaged frozen salmon fillets and thaw them before use. You can also make this with a 6-ounce can of salmon (well drained) or smoked salmon.

Per serving: Calories: 226; Total Fat: 18g; Total Carbs: 1g; Fiber: 0g; Net Carbs: 1g; Protein: 15g
Macronutrients: Fat: 71%; Protein: 28%; Carbs: 1%

Keto Blueberry Pancakes

Makes 12
Prep time: 10 minutes

Cook time: 20 minutes
Total time: 30 minutes

Just because you're eating a keto diet doesn't mean you can't enjoy this breakfast staple. Finely ground almond flour from blanched almonds makes a great substitute for wheat flour. The small number of blueberries provide flavor and nutrition without adding too many carbs from the natural fruit sugars. These are easily refrigerated (or frozen) and reheated in the microwave or warmed in a skillet over low heat. Be sure to use finely ground blanched almond flour—my favorite brand is Bob's Red Mill— because almond meal results in a gritty, mealy texture that most people don't enjoy.

2½ cups finely ground blanched almond flour, sifted
2 teaspoons baking powder
4 eggs, lightly beaten
⅔ cup almond milk

½ cup butter, melted, plus more for serving
1 teaspoon vanilla extract
½ cup fresh blueberries
Nonstick cooking spray
Sugar-free pancake syrup (optional)

1. In a large bowl, whisk the flour and baking powder until evenly combined.

2. Add the eggs, almond milk, butter, and vanilla and whisk until smooth. Carefully fold in the blueberries.

3. Preheat a nonstick skillet or griddle over medium-high heat, and coat with cooking spray or brush lightly with oil.

4. Using a dry measuring cup, pour ¼ cup of batter into the skillet for each pancake. (You'll cook in batches.)

5. When bubbles start to appear on the surface of the pancakes, carefully flip. (Only flip once to maintain fluffiness.)

6. Cook for 2 to 3 minutes more, then transfer to a plate. Repeat with the remaining batter.

7. Serve topped with melted butter and/or your favorite brand of sugar-free pancake syrup (if using).

SUBSTITUTION TIP: Swap out the blueberries for sugar-free chocolate chips.

Per serving: Calories: 387; Total Fat: 35g; Total Carbs: 12g; Fiber: 4g; Net Carbs: 8g; Protein: 11g
Macronutrients: Fat: 77%; Protein: 12%; Carbs: 11%

Ham and Cheese Egg Cups

Makes 12   **Cook time:** 20 minutes
Prep time: 5 minutes   **Total time:** 25 minutes

These ham and cheese egg cups are very simple but make a beautiful presentation with a poached whole egg. Deli ham becomes a delicious cup with crispy edges that holds a perfectly cooked egg atop a bed of melted cheese. If you plan to serve these all at once for a crowd, cook them to your desired egg consistency. If you plan to batch cook these for enjoying over several days, it's best to bake them until the yolk is fully cooked. They are great cold or reheated in the microwave.

Nonstick cooking spray
12 slices deli ham (about 1 pound)
1 cup shredded cheddar cheese
12 eggs

Salt
Freshly ground black pepper
Paprika (optional)
2 or 3 scallions (green parts only), sliced

1. Preheat the oven to 400°F.

2. Lightly spray a muffin tin with cooking spray.

3. Place a slice of ham over each muffin cup and press down to form a cup shape.

4. Evenly divide the cheese between the 12 cups.

5. Carefully crack 1 egg into each cup, keeping the yolk intact.

6. Lightly season with salt, pepper, and a pinch of paprika (if using).

7. Bake for 18 minutes or until the yolks are done to your liking.

8. While still hot, garnish with the scallions, then allow to cool slightly before serving. (The eggs will continue to cook for a few minutes after removing them from the oven.) Store in an airtight container with a piece of parchment paper between the layers.

Per serving: Calories: 172; Total Fat: 11g; Total Carbs: 2g; Fiber: 1g; Net Carbs: 1g; Protein: 15g
Macronutrients: Fat: 59%; Protein: 37%; Carbs: 4%

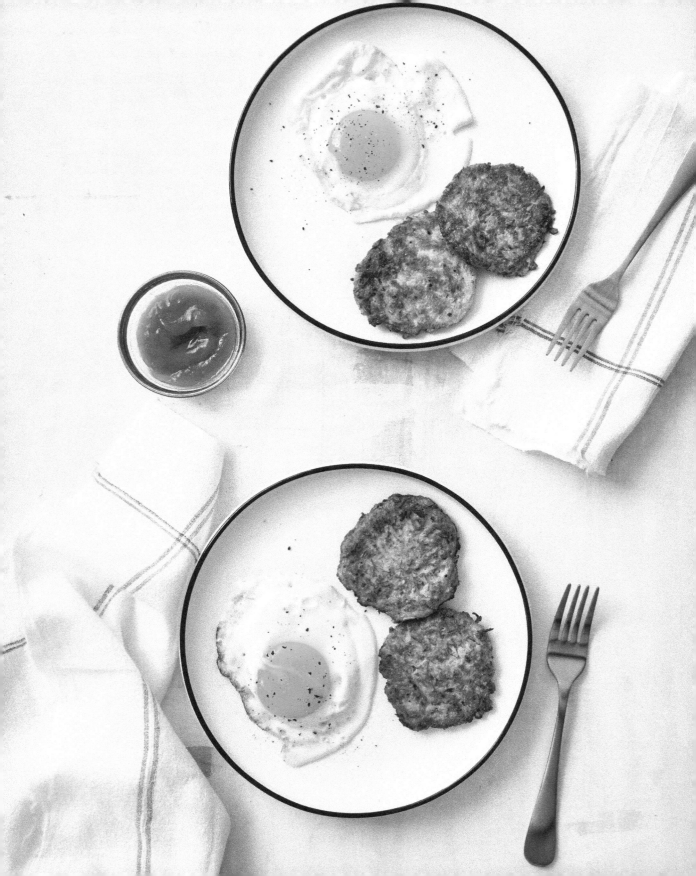

Classic Diner Hash Browns

SUPER SAVER

Serves 6
Prep time: 10 minutes

Cook time: 30 minutes
Total time: 40 minutes

Just because you can't eat potatoes doesn't mean you have to miss out on crispy hash browns. These are made keto friendly with radishes. These peppery little vegetables really mellow when cooked and become very potato-like. The trick to re-creating the crispy, beautifully browned edges of a "real" hash brown is to remove as much water as possible. These hash browns are delicious served with fried eggs and a bit of sugar-free ketchup.

3 cups radishes
2 eggs
½ cup finely shredded Parmesan cheese

½ teaspoon salt
½ teaspoon freshly ground black pepper
Nonstick cooking spray or oil

1. Preheat the oven to its lowest setting possible.

2. Using a box grater or the grating blade of a food processor, grate the radishes. (No need to peel them.)

3. Place the radishes in a microwave-safe bowl with a plate on top, and microwave at full power for 3 minutes. Allow to cool.

4. Turn out the cooled radishes onto a clean tea towel or cheesecloth and squeeze well to remove as much liquid as possible. Discard the liquid and return the radishes to the bowl.

5. Add the eggs, cheese, salt, and pepper, and mix well with a fork.

6. Preheat a nonstick skillet over medium-high heat. Coat the skillet with cooking spray.

7. In batches of two, form the radish mixture into patties and flatten as thin as possible.

8. Cook over medium heat for 4 to 5 minutes per side or until the patties are browned and crisp. Transfer to a baking sheet and place in the oven while you continue cooking in batches. Wipe the skillet with a paper towel and reapply cooking spray between each batch.

9. Serve immediately.

Per serving: Calories: 68; Total Fat: 4g; Total Carbs: 3g; Fiber: 1g; Net Carbs: 2g; Protein: 5g
Macronutrients: Fat: 52%; Protein: 30%; Carbs: 18%

Baked Egg Avocado Boats

Makes 6
Prep time: 10 minutes

Cook time: 15 minutes
Total time: 25 minutes

The creaminess of this dish is its absolute appeal. The softness of the avocado with the slightly runny yolk of a perfect oven-poached egg is a delicious combination. Eggs are a great budget-friendly protein source, and the avocado provides an abundance of fiber and healthy fat. (Avocados are particularly affordable in the spring and summer when California's avocado crops come to market.)

Nonstick cooking spray
3 large ripe avocados, halved and pitted
6 eggs

Salt
Freshly ground black pepper
2 tablespoons salsa (optional)

1. Preheat the oven to 425°F. Lightly spray a baking sheet with cooking spray. (Or lightly coat the baking sheet with oil or line it with parchment paper.)

2. Use a small spoon to scoop out just enough of the avocado flesh to hold 1 egg in the cavity. Put the removed avocado in a small bowl.

3. Arrange the avocado halves faceup on the baking sheet.

4. Carefully crack an egg into each avocado half, keeping the yolk intact. Season lightly with salt and pepper.

5. Bake for about 15 minutes or until the egg yolks are done to your liking.

6. Allow to cool slightly. (The eggs will continue to cook for a few minutes after removing them from the oven.)

7. With a fork, mash the reserved avocado flesh, mix it with the salsa (if using), and serve alongside as a garnish.

> BATCH-COOKING TIP: These boats are best eaten fresh out of the oven and don't store well. But as you can see, it's easy to use just 1 avocado and 2 eggs when serving breakfast for two.

Per serving: Calories: 254; Total Fat: 20g; Total Carbs: 12g; Fiber: 9g; Net Carbs: 3g; Protein: 10g
Macronutrients: Fat: 67%; Protein: 16%; Carbs: 17%

Cheesy Sausage and Cabbage Hash

Serves 6
Prep time: 10 minutes

Cook time: 25 minutes
Total time: 35 minutes

Cabbage for breakfast? You bet! The high fiber content of cabbage is filling and a great way to start the day. Cabbage is also budget friendly because it keeps very well in the refrigerator, and a large head goes a long way. You can use red or green, but red cabbage provides additional nutrition from the heart-healthy anthocyanins that give it the red color. If you have bacon fat on hand, be sure to use it instead of olive oil for an extra kick of flavor. This dish is great fresh out of the oven and is also just as good reheated the next day. If you're extra hungry, serve it alongside a fried egg.

---

2 tablespoons olive oil or bacon fat
½ cup diced onion
1 garlic clove, minced
1½ pounds kielbasa sausage, cut into
  1-inch rounds

4 cups chopped red or green cabbage
½ teaspoon salt
½ teaspoon freshly ground black pepper
1½ cups shredded cheddar cheese

1. Preheat the oven to 400°F.

2. Warm the oil in a large skillet over medium heat, then add the onion and garlic. Cook, while stirring, for 1 to 2 minutes until fragrant. (Keep it moving so the garlic does not burn.)

3. Add the kielbasa and brown for 5 minutes, stirring regularly.

4. Add the cabbage, salt, and pepper, and sauté for 8 to 10 minutes, stirring regularly.

5. If your skillet is oven safe (e.g., cast iron or stainless steel), you can use it for the remaining steps. If it is not oven safe (e.g., it has a plastic handle), transfer the mixture to a 9-by-13-inch glass baking dish.

6. Top the cabbage-and-sausage mixture with the cheese.

7. Bake for 10 minutes. Turn the broiler to high for the last minute to ensure the cheese is melted. Remove from the oven and serve.

Per serving: Calories: 547; Total Fat: 48g; Total Carbs: 10g; Fiber: 2g; Net Carbs: 8g; Protein: 20g
Macronutrients: Fat: 78%; Protein: 14%; Carbs: 8%

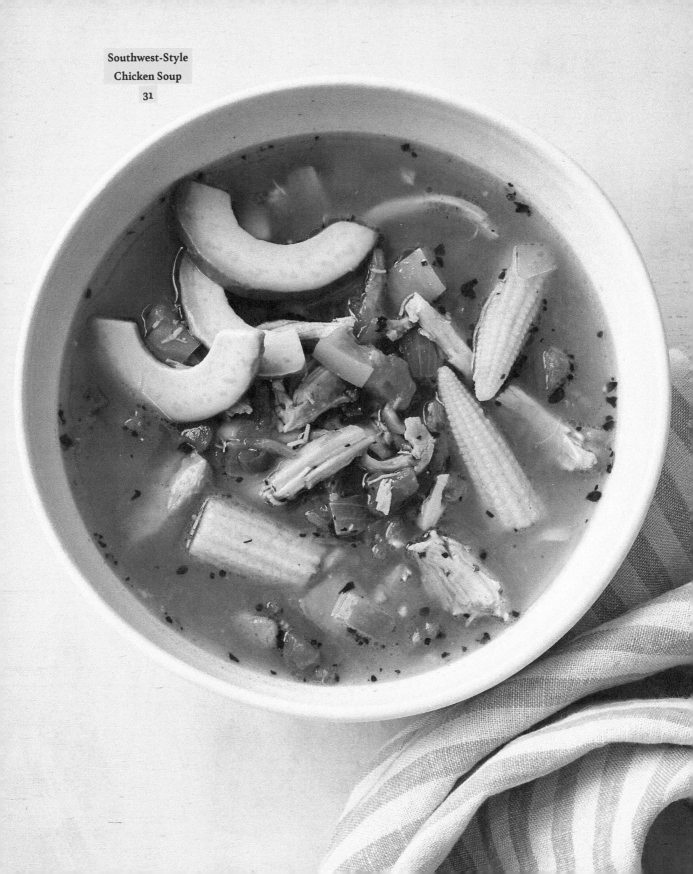

CHAPTER 3

Soups and Salads

Chicken and Baby Corn
Chowder 28

Creamy Keto Seafood Stew 30

Southwest-Style Chicken
Soup 31

Broccoli Cheddar Soup 32

Zuppa Toscana (Sausage and
Kale Soup) 33

Keto Beef Chili 35

Creamy Dill and Radish
"Potato" Salad 36

Classic Chicken Salad 37

Classic Tuna Salad 38

Spinach Salad with Warm
Bacon Dressing 39

Classic Cobb Salad 41

Cool and Creamy Cucumber
Tomato Salad 42

Chicken and Baby Corn Chowder

Serves 6 to 8
Prep time: 10 minutes

Cook time: 1 hour
Total time: 1 hour 10 minutes

Creamy chicken chowder dotted with plump corn kernels is a textural delight, one that is hard to replicate on keto. Then I discovered canned baby corn. It has a very low carb count because it hasn't matured and developed the starches found in ripe corn. It doesn't have a lot of flavor, but it does have that familiar corn texture if you chop it into corn kernel–size pieces. Baby corn is usually found in the Asian food aisle of the supermarket alongside bamboo shoots and water chestnuts. Despite its many ingredients, this recipe comes together quickly and is great for portioning and freezing for a rainy "comfort food" day.

½ pound bacon, cut into 1-inch slices
2 pounds boneless, skinless chicken
    thighs, diced
3 tablespoons butter
1 medium white onion, diced
3 garlic cloves, minced
1 red bell pepper, diced
1 cup diced cauliflower florets
6 cups low-sodium chicken broth, divided

2 (15-ounce) cans baby corn, drained
    and chopped
1 teaspoon salt
1 teaspoon freshly ground black pepper
1½ cups heavy cream
8 ounces full-fat cream cheese, cubed, at
    room temperature
2 or 3 scallions, sliced

1. In a large soup pot over medium heat, brown the bacon for 5 to 7 minutes or until crispy. Using a slotted spoon or fork, transfer the bacon to a paper towel.

2. In the bacon fat, cook the chicken until cooked through. Remove from the pan and set aside.

3. Add the butter to the remaining fat, along with the onion, garlic, bell pepper, and cauliflower. Cook for about 8 minutes or until the onion starts to become translucent.

4. Add 1 cup of broth and use a wooden spoon to scrape the bottom of the pot to deglaze.

5. Return the chicken to the pot and add the remaining 5 cups of broth, baby corn, salt, and pepper. Turn up the heat to high and stir well to combine.

6. When the soup is almost at a boil, turn the heat down to low, cover, and simmer for 30 to 35 minutes. Stir regularly, making sure to scrape the bottom of the pot to prevent sticking.

7. Remove the pot from the heat and add the cream and cream cheese. Stir well to melt. (Adding these at the end prevents the cream from separating and ruining the chowder.)

8. Taste for seasoning. Depending on the amount of sodium in your broth, you may need additional salt.

9. Serve in large bowls, garnished with the bacon and scallions.

METHOD TIP: To make this in a multicooker, follow the recipe as written but use the Sauté setting for the bacon, chicken, and vegetable steps. Add about a cup of broth and use a wooden spoon to scrape the bottom and deglaze the pot. Add the remaining broth and other ingredients (except the cream and cream cheese). Secure the lid and cook on low pressure for 20 minutes, using a quick release at the end of the cook time. Carefully open the lid, stir in the cream and cream cheese off the heat, and serve.

Per serving: Calories: 846; Total Fat: 64g; Total Carbs: 24g; Fiber: 4g; Net Carbs: 20g; Protein: 45g
Macronutrients: Fat: 67%; Protein: 22%; Carbs: 11%

Creamy Keto Seafood Stew

Serves 6
Prep time: 10 minutes

Cook time: 30 minutes
Total time: 40 minutes

This creamy chowder tastes authentic without budget-busting fresh seafood. By using affordable canned seafood (shrimp, clams, and crab), you can achieve a similar depth of flavor at a fraction of the cost.

½ pound bacon, cut into 1-inch slices
½ medium white onion, diced
2 celery stalks, diced
3 garlic cloves, minced
2 cups frozen cauliflower rice
1 teaspoon salt
2 teaspoons freshly ground black pepper
3 cups low-sodium chicken broth

1 (8-ounce) jar clam juice
1 (6-ounce) can medium shrimp, drained
1 (6-ounce) can crabmeat, with juices
1 (10-ounce) can chopped clams, with juices
1½ cups heavy cream
8 ounces full-fat cream cheese, cubed, at room temperature
½ cup shredded cheddar cheese

1. In a large soup pot over medium heat, brown the bacon for 5 to 7 minutes or until crispy. Using a slotted spoon or fork, transfer the bacon to a paper towel.

2. Pour off all but 2 tablespoons of the fat. Raise the heat to medium-high.

3. Add the onion, celery, garlic, cauliflower rice, salt, and pepper. Sauté until the vegetables are soft, about 10 minutes. Stir frequently to prevent the garlic from burning.

4. Add the chicken broth and use a wooden spoon to scrape the bottom of the pot to deglaze. Lower the heat to medium and allow to simmer for 15 minutes to continue to soften the vegetables.

5. Turn the heat to low and add the clam juice and shrimp along with the crabmeat and clams with their canning liquid. Stir to combine.

6. Add the cream and cream cheese. Stir to melt the cream cheese and allow to sit, covered, on low heat for a few minutes to meld.

7. Stir well and taste for seasoning. Serve in bowls, garnished with the bacon and cheddar.

METHOD TIP: If you like your stew even thicker, before you add the seafood and dairy, use an immersion stick blender to puree the soup a bit.

Per serving: Calories: 662; Total Fat: 55g; Total Carbs: 11g; Fiber: 1g; Net Carbs: 10g; Protein: 32g
Macronutrients: Fat: 74%; Protein: 20%; Carbs: 6%

Southwest-Style Chicken Soup

Serves 6
Prep time: 10 minutes

Cook time: 55 minutes
Total time: 1 hour 5 minutes

The diced tomatoes and green chiles lend a familiar Southwest flavor to this hearty chicken soup, and if you're curious how baby corn fits into a keto diet, check out the headnote for the Chicken and Baby Corn Chowder recipe on page 28.

2 tablespoons olive oil
1 medium white onion, diced
1 bell pepper, diced
1 jalapeño pepper, seeded and diced
3 garlic cloves, minced
1 tablespoon chili powder
1 teaspoon ground cumin
1 teaspoon dried oregano
1 teaspoon salt
1 teaspoon freshly ground black pepper

6 cups low-sodium chicken broth, divided
2 pounds boneless, skinless chicken thighs
1 (10-ounce) can tomatoes and green chiles (such as Ro-Tel brand)
4 ounces full-fat cream cheese, cubed, at room temperature
1 (15-ounce) can baby corn, drained and chopped
1 cup shredded cheddar cheese
1 avocado, pitted and sliced

1. In a large soup pot over medium-high heat, heat the oil.

2. Add the onion, bell pepper, jalapeño, and garlic. Sauté for 6 to 8 minutes or until the onion becomes translucent.

3. Add the chili powder, cumin, oregano, salt, and pepper, and stir until fragrant, 1 to 2 minutes.

4. Add 1 cup of broth to the pot and scrape the bottom with a wooden spoon to deglaze.

5. Add the chicken thighs, pour in the remaining 5 cups of broth, and add the tomatoes and green chiles.

6. Raise the heat to high. When the soup just comes to a boil, lower the heat to medium-low, cover, and cook for 45 minutes.

7. Transfer the chicken to a cutting board. Using two forks, shred the meat and return it to the pot.

8. Remove the pot from the heat and stir in the cream cheese and baby corn. Stir well to melt the cheese. Allow to sit for 10 minutes to combine.

9. Serve in large bowls, garnished with the cheddar and avocado.

Per serving: Calories: 524; Total Fat: 31g; Total Carbs: 23g; Fiber: 7g; Net Carbs: 16g; Protein: 44g
Macronutrients: Fat: 52%; Protein: 33%; Carbs: 15%

Broccoli Cheddar Soup

Serves 6
Prep time: 10 minutes

Cook time: 20 minutes
Total time: 30 minutes

There is nothing better on a cold day than a big bowl of broccoli cheddar soup. If you don't have fresh broccoli on hand, frozen broccoli florets will work. They'll need to be thawed and chopped, and the color won't be as vibrantly green as with fresh broccoli, but the flavor will still be great.

---

8 tablespoons butter
½ medium white onion, diced
2 celery stalks, diced
2 garlic cloves, minced
4 cups diced broccoli florets
6 cups low-sodium chicken broth
1 cup heavy cream

4 ounces full-fat cream cheese, cubed,
　at room temperature
16 ounces sharp cheddar cheese, freshly
　grated, plus more for garnish
Salt
Freshly ground black pepper

1. In a large stockpot over medium heat, melt the butter.

2. Add the onion, celery, and garlic, and sauté until the onion is soft and translucent, 8 to 10 minutes.

3. Add the broccoli and cook for 5 minutes until the broccoli is vibrantly green and soft.

4. Remove about ½ cup of broccoli and set aside for garnish.

5. Add the broth and cream. While stirring, bring to a gentle boil then immediately lower the heat to low.

6. Add the cream cheese and stir.

7. Slowly add small amounts of cheddar, stirring constantly. Continue until all the cheese has been incorporated. Add salt and pepper to taste.

8. Divide between bowls and garnish with the reserved broccoli and additional cheddar.

> **INGREDIENT TIP:** Many packaged shredded cheeses have a small amount of cellulose or other anticaking agents that prevent the shreds from sticking together in the bag. These can prevent the cheese from properly melting into the soup. Skip the bag for this recipe and freshly grate a block; it's usually cheaper, anyway.

Per serving: Calories: 703; Total Fat: 63g; Total Carbs: 11g; Fiber: 2g; Net Carbs: 9g; Protein: 26g
Macronutrients: Fat: 80%; Protein: 14%; Carbs: 6%

Zuppa Toscana (Sausage and Kale Soup)

Serves 6
Prep time: 10 minutes

Cook time: 45 minutes
Total time: 55 minutes

This classic comfort soup is bright and cheerful any time of the year, but especially when it's cold outside. This keto version removes the traditional potatoes and uses cauliflower instead. Kale adds a nutritional boost, but you can easily replace it with baby spinach. The Parmesan cheese is the perfect garnish to this delicious, broth-based soup.

½ pound bacon, cut into 1-inch slices
1 pound hot Italian sausage, casings removed
1 medium onion, diced
3 garlic cloves, minced
6 cups low-sodium chicken broth

1 head cauliflower, stemmed and chopped
3 cups stemmed and chopped kale or
   baby spinach
½ cup heavy cream
½ cup shredded Parmesan cheese

1. In a large soup pot over medium-high heat, brown the bacon for 5 to 7 minutes or until crispy. Using a slotted spoon or fork, transfer the bacon to a paper towel.

2. Pour off all but 2 tablespoons of the fat. Lower the heat to medium.

3. Add the sausage to the pot and cook until browned, about 5 minutes. Break up the sausage with the spoon.

4. Add the onion and garlic and sauté until the onions are translucent, about 7 minutes. Stir frequently to prevent the garlic from burning.

5. Add the broth. Use a wooden spoon to scrape the bottom of the pot to deglaze. Cover and simmer for 10 minutes.

6. Add the cauliflower. Cover and simmer for 10 minutes or until the cauliflower is soft.

7. Add the kale, cream, and reserved bacon, and simmer for 5 minutes to allow the kale to wilt.

8. Serve in large bowls, garnished with the Parmesan.

METHOD TIP: To make this soup in a multicooker, follow the recipe as written but use the Sauté setting for the bacon, sausage, and vegetable steps. Add about a cup of broth, and use a wooden spoon to scrape the bottom and deglaze the pot. Add the remaining broth and other ingredients (except the cream and kale). Secure the lid and cook on low pressure for 15 minutes, using a quick release at the end of the cook time. Afterward, use the Sauté setting for 5 minutes while stirring in the cream and kale.

Per serving: Calories: 493; Total Fat: 40g; Total Carbs: 10g; Fiber: 2g; Net Carbs: 8g; Protein: 24g
Macronutrients: Fat: 72%; Protein: 20%; Carbs: 8%

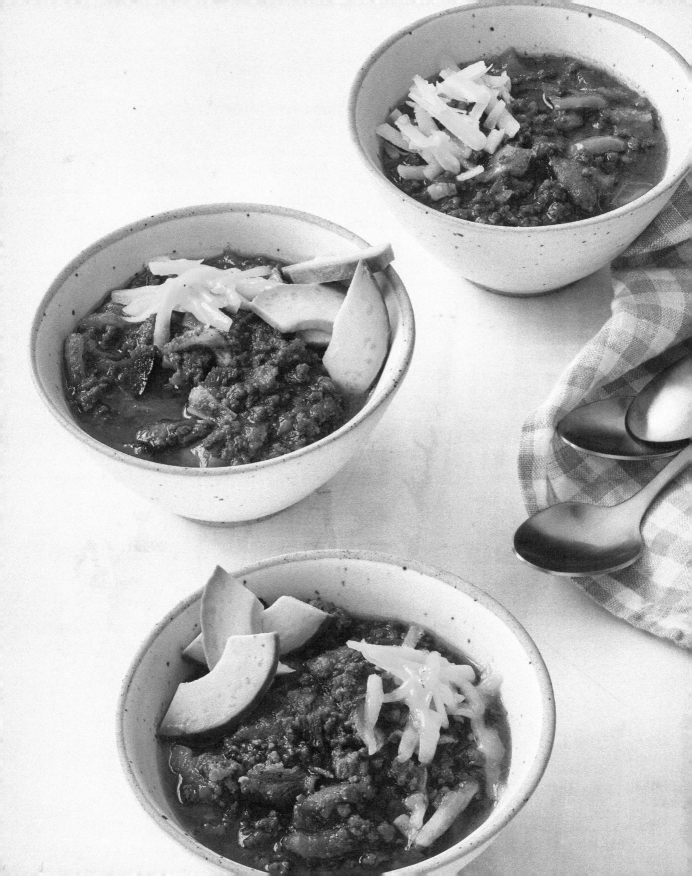

Keto Beef Chili

Serves 8
Prep time: 10 minutes

Cook time: 1 hour
Total time: 1 hour 10 minutes

Beef chili is a family favorite in many homes. This version cuts out the beans (which many chili aficionados would say don't belong, anyway) and uses less tomato to help cut down on natural sugars. I'm willing to bet that you won't be able to tell the difference between this recipe and your favorite non-keto chili. Pile it high with sliced avocado, sour cream, and shredded cheese for the perfect cool and creamy complements.

2 pounds ground beef
3 slices bacon, diced
1 medium white onion, diced
1 red bell pepper, diced
1 jalapeño, seeded and diced
3 garlic cloves, minced
1 (6-ounce) can tomato paste
3 tablespoons chili powder
2 teaspoons ground cumin

1 teaspoon salt
1 teaspoon freshly ground black pepper
3 or 4 dashes hot sauce (optional)
1 (15-ounce) can diced tomatoes
3 cups low-sodium beef broth, store bought or homemade (page 122)
1 avocado, pitted and sliced
½ cup sour cream
1 cup shredded cheddar cheese

1. In a large soup pot over medium heat, cook the beef, bacon, onion, bell pepper, jalapeño, and garlic until the beef is browned. Drain the excess fat from the pot.

2. Add the tomato paste, chili powder, cumin, salt, pepper, and hot sauce (if using), and cook until the spices become fragrant, about 5 minutes.

3. Add the diced tomatoes and broth, scraping the bottom of the pot with a wooden spoon to deglaze. Increase the heat to high and bring to a gentle boil. Reduce the heat to medium-low and simmer, uncovered, for 45 minutes.

4. Serve in large bowls, garnished with the avocado, sour cream, and cheddar.

Per serving: Calories: 502; Total Fat: 37g; Total Carbs: 15g; Fiber: 6g; Net Carbs: 9g; Protein: 30g
Macronutrients: Fat: 66%; Protein: 24%; Carbs: 10%

Creamy Dill and Radish "Potato" Salad

Serves 6
Prep time: 10 minutes

Cook time: 10 minutes, plus 1 hour to overnight for chilling

Total time: 1 hour 20 minutes

This salad is as beautiful as it is delicious. The "faux-tato" substitute is red radishes. When boiled and drained, most of the peppery spiciness of raw radishes is removed, leaving you with a mellow vegetable that mimics the flavor of potatoes. The dill in this salad adds a delicate herbal freshness that will make your friends and family sit up and take notice. Be sure your radishes are completely dry before mixing them into the dressing. Many people like warm potato salad, but I think this salad is best when it's been in the refrigerator overnight.

5 cups red radishes
½ cup mayonnaise
½ cup diced celery
2 dill pickles, diced
⅓ cup minced red onion
3 tablespoons chopped fresh dill or
  1 tablespoon dried

2 teaspoons Dijon mustard
Juice of ½ lemon (1 tablespoon)
½ teaspoon salt
½ teaspoon freshly ground black pepper
2 hard-boiled eggs, peeled and chopped

1. Wash the radishes, cut off the tops and bottoms, and cut in half or quarters, for roughly 1½-inch pieces.

2. Place the radishes in a shallow pan with just enough to water to cover. Bring to a boil, reduce the heat to low, cover, and simmer for 5 minutes.

3. Drain the radishes and turn them out onto folded paper towels or a tea towel to cool and dry completely.

4. In a large bowl, stir together the mayonnaise, celery, pickles, onion, dill, mustard, lemon juice, salt, and pepper.

5. Use a paper towel to dry the radishes thoroughly. Add the radishes and eggs to the bowl and gently fold into the dressing.

6. Refrigerate for at least 1 hour (preferably overnight) and serve chilled.

INGREDIENT TIP: Make sure to find a brand of mayonnaise without added sugar. Two of my favorites are Primal Kitchen Avocado Oil Mayonnaise and Duke's Real Mayonnaise.

Per serving: Calories: 174; Total Fat: 16g; Total Carbs: 6g; Fiber: 2g; Net Carbs: 4g; Protein: 3g
Macronutrients: Fat: 81%; Protein: 7%; Carbs: 12%

Classic Chicken Salad

Serves 6   **Total time:** 1 hour 10 minutes

Prep time: 10 minutes, plus 1 hour to
overnight for chilling

Creamy chicken salad is a staple for a reason. It is delicious, stores well, is easy to make in large batches, and can be served numerous ways. It's also a great way to use leftover chicken. One way to keep this dish budget friendly is to use a day-old rotisserie chicken, which can often be purchased for half price in the cold section of the grocery deli. Another great option is canned chicken.

3 cups chopped cooked chicken
2 scallions, sliced
1 celery stalk, thinly sliced
1 teaspoon Dijon mustard
½ cup plus 2 tablespoons mayonnaise

½ teaspoon salt
½ teaspoon freshly ground black pepper
¼ cup slivered almonds (optional)
Lettuce, for serving (optional)

1. In a large bowl, combine all the ingredients. Mix well.

2. Refrigerate for at least 1 hour (preferably overnight for best flavor).

3. Serve as is, in a lettuce cup, or on a bed of salad greens.

Per serving: Calories: 266; Total Fat: 20g; Total Carbs: 1g; Fiber: 0g; Net Carbs: 1g; Protein: 19g
Macronutrients: Fat: 69%; Protein: 30%; Carbs: 1%

Classic Tuna Salad

Serves 6

Total time: 1 hour 10 minutes

Prep time: 10 minutes, plus 1 hour to overnight for chilling

The texture and flavor of oil-packed tuna is far superior to the water-packed version, and you get the added benefit of the heart-healthy olive oil that remains behind after it's drained. Like the Classic Chicken Salad (page 37), this salad also improves with some time chilling out in the refrigerator.

3 (5-ounce) cans tuna packed in olive oil, drained
2 hard-boiled eggs, peeled and chopped
2 scallions, sliced
1 celery stalk, thinly sliced
1 tablespoon sugar-free pickle relish (I like Mt. Olive brand)

1 teaspoon Dijon mustard
½ cup plus 2 tablespoons mayonnaise
½ teaspoon salt
½ teaspoon freshly ground black pepper
2 to 4 dashes hot sauce (optional)
Lettuce, for serving (optional)

1. In a large bowl, combine all the ingredients. Mix well.

2. Refrigerate for 1 hour (preferably overnight for best flavor).

3. Serve as is, in a lettuce cup, or on a bed of salad greens.

SUBSTITUTION TIP: Swap out the canned tuna for a 15-ounce can of pink salmon to make a delicious salmon salad.

Per serving: Calories: 292; Total Fat: 23g; Total Carbs: 2g; Fiber: 0g; Net Carbs: 2g; Protein: 17g
Macronutrients: Fat: 72%; Protein: 26%; Carbs: 2%

Spinach Salad with Warm Bacon Dressing

Serves 6
Prep time: 10 minutes

Cook time: 25 minutes
Total time: 35 minutes

A warm dressing on cool greens probably sounds like an unusual combination, but this might become one of your favorite salads. To make the dressing lightly sweet, I use a small amount of erythritol-based sweetener. The warm bacon fat helps it dissolve, and it's the perfect complement to tangy red wine vinegar. (See page 5 for where to purchase erythritol sweeteners at bargain prices.)

12 bacon slices
5 tablespoons red wine vinegar
1 teaspoon erythritol-based sweetener
1 teaspoon Dijon mustard
¼ teaspoon salt

¼ teaspoon freshly ground black pepper
12 ounces baby spinach
4 hard-boiled eggs, peeled and sliced
6 large button mushrooms, thinly sliced
1 small red onion, very thinly sliced

1. Cook the bacon in a skillet or using the baking sheet method on page 41, chop, and set aside.

2. Transfer 4 tablespoons of bacon fat to a small saucepan over low heat.

3. Add the vinegar, sweetener, mustard, salt, and pepper.

4. Whisk vigorously until a vinaigrette is formed and the sweetener is dissolved. Let it sit over low heat to stay warm.

5. In a large salad bowl, gently toss together the spinach, eggs, mushrooms, onion, and bacon.

6. When ready to serve, drizzle the hot vinaigrette over the salad and toss again. Serve immediately.

BATCH-COOKING TIP: If you'll be making this salad ahead, toss the ingredients and store in a covered container in the refrigerator. Put the dressing in a bowl, cover with plastic wrap, and store in the refrigerator. Warm up the dressing in the microwave just before serving.

Per serving: Calories: 162; Total Fat: 11g; Total Carbs: 4g; Fiber: 2g; Net Carbs: 2g; Protein: 12g; Erythritol: 1g
Macronutrients: Fat: 60%; Protein: 31%; Carbs: 9%

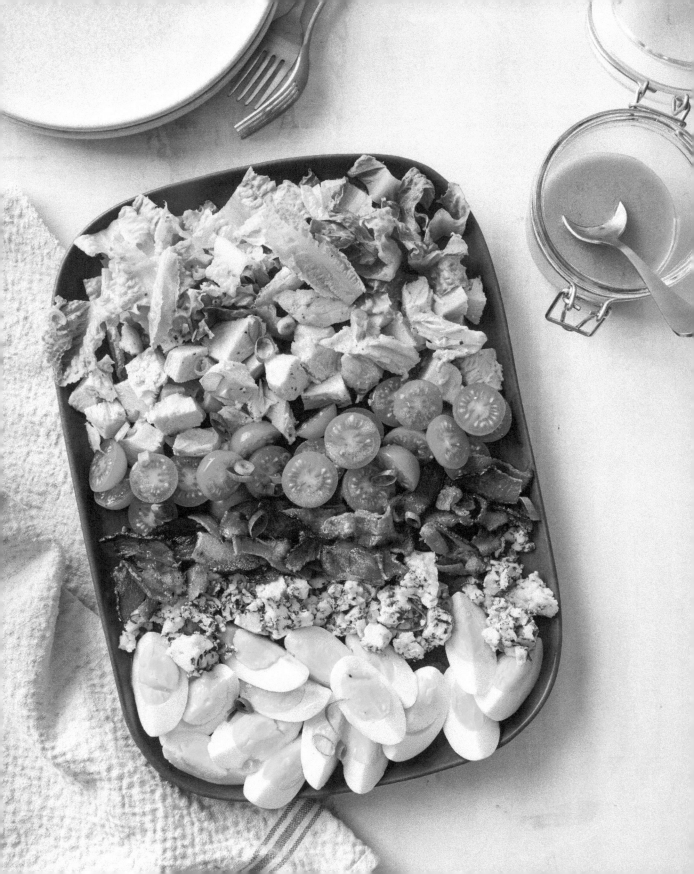

Classic Cobb Salad

Serves 6
Prep time: 20 minutes

Total time: 20 minutes

Cobb salad is a classic American dish filled with an array of fresh ingredients that come together in the most perfect way—and it also happens to be keto without even trying! A leftover, cold rotisserie chicken is perfect for the protein. Cooking the bacon on a baking sheet in the oven at 375°F for 25 minutes (or until crisp) makes for easy cleanup, perfectly flat bacon, and beautifully rendered bacon fat for future recipes. If you want to prep this salad once to eat over the next few days, keep the dressing in a sealed jar. Lightly sprinkle lemon juice on the avocado slices and store in an airtight container.

¼ cup red wine vinegar
⅓ cup extra-virgin olive oil
1 tablespoon Dijon mustard
¼ teaspoon salt
¼ teaspoon freshly ground black pepper
1 large head romaine lettuce, chopped
1 pound cooked chicken, chopped

10 strips cooked bacon, crumbled
6 hard-boiled eggs, peeled and sliced
6 ounces cherry tomatoes, halved
1 avocado, pitted and sliced
6 ounces blue cheese crumbles
3 scallions, sliced

1. To make the dressing, combine the vinegar, oil, mustard, salt, and pepper in a jar with a lid and shake vigorously.

2. Spread the lettuce in a large salad bowl or platter.

3. Making rows across the lettuce, arrange the chicken, bacon, eggs, tomatoes, avocado, and blue cheese.

4. Drizzle the dressing over the salad and garnish with the scallions.

Per serving: Calories: 496; Total Fat: 52g; Total Carbs: 10g; Fiber: 6g; Net Carbs: 4g; Protein: 40g
Macronutrients: Fat: 60%; Protein: 34%; Carbs: 6%

Cool and Creamy Cucumber Tomato Salad

Serves 6

Prep time: 15 minutes, plus 1 hour to overnight to chill

Total time: 1 hour 15 minutes

Everyone is familiar with the coleslaws and potato salads that fill the tables of family gatherings and barbecues. This salad is a welcome change. The sweet, creamy dressing cuts through the spiciness of the red onion and helps maintain the crunchy texture of the cucumbers—even after several days in the refrigerator. This needs to chill for at least an hour before serving, but as is the case with many recipes in this book, it gets even better overnight. Just gently toss again before serving.

¾ cup mayonnaise
2 tablespoons white vinegar
2 teaspoons erythritol-based sweetener
½ teaspoon salt

½ teaspoon freshly ground black pepper
5 large cucumbers, peeled and thinly sliced
1 small red onion, halved and thinly sliced
5 ounces cherry tomatoes, halved

1. In a large bowl, whisk together the mayonnaise, vinegar, sweetener, salt, and pepper.

2. Add the cucumbers, onion, and tomatoes. Gently toss to coat.

3. Chill for at least 1 hour (preferably overnight).

4. Gently toss again before serving.

Per serving: Calories: 234; Total Fat: 21g; Total Carbs: 11g; Fiber: 2g; Net Carbs: 9g; Protein: 2g; Erythritol: 1g
Macronutrients: Fat: 80%; Protein: 3%; Carbs: 17%

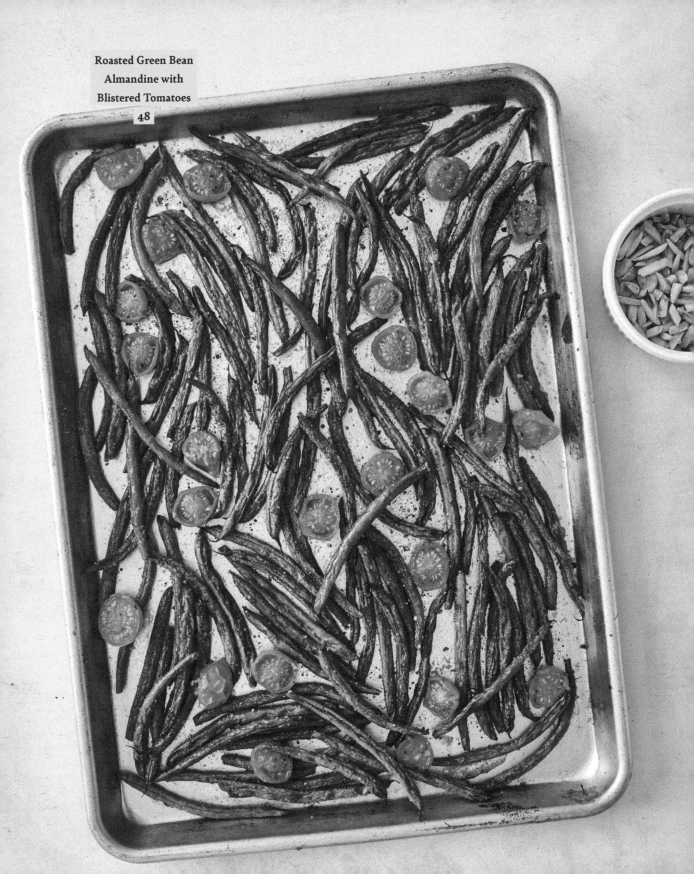

Roasted Green Bean
Almandine with
Blistered Tomatoes

48

CHAPTER 4

Vegetables

Italian Zucchini Boats 46

Bacon-Wrapped
Asparagus 47

Roasted Green Bean
Almandine with Blistered
Tomatoes 48

Loaded Mashed
Cauliflower 49

Crispy Pan-Roasted
Broccoli 51

Easy Cauliflower Rice 52

Zucchini Noodles 53

Roasted Cabbage Steaks 55

Pan-Roasted Red Radish
"Potatoes" 56

Creamed Spinach 57

Southern-Style Collard
Greens 58

Crispy Pan-Roasted Okra 59

Italian Zucchini Boats

Serves 6
Prep time: 10 minutes

Cook time: 20 minutes
Total time: 30 minutes

This recipe is great as a side dish but can be hearty enough for a main dish if you serve two zucchini halves alongside a big salad. Be sure to use a low-carb marinara sauce without added sugar. Most major brands have lots of additional carbs. I really enjoy Rao's Homemade Marinara Sauce, but it can be pricey. The Silver Palate brand and Great Value lines by Walmart both have no-sugar marinara sauces at more affordable prices.

3 large zucchini squash
1 tablespoon olive oil
½ pound mild Italian sausage, casings removed
½ teaspoon onion powder
½ teaspoon garlic powder

½ teaspoon dried oregano or Italian seasoning
½ teaspoon salt
½ teaspoon freshly ground black pepper
1 cup sugar-free marinara sauce
1 cup shredded mozzarella cheese

1. Preheat the oven to 375°F.
2. Slice the zucchini in half lengthwise. Use the tip of a spoon to scrape out the center, leaving the skin and a small layer of flesh intact. Coarsely chop the removed zucchini flesh and reserve.
3. Lightly oil a 9-by-13-inch casserole pan and arrange the zucchini "boats" cut-side up.
4. In a large skillet over medium heat, brown the sausage while breaking it up with a spoon. Drain off any excess oil.
5. Add the reserved zucchini flesh, onion powder, garlic powder, oregano, salt, and pepper. Cook for 6 to 8 minutes or until the zucchini is tender.
6. Using a slotted spoon, evenly divide the sausage and zucchini mixture into the 6 zucchini boats, leaving behind any extra liquid.
7. Evenly spoon the marinara sauce over the stuffed zucchini boats. Top with the mozzarella.
8. Bake for 8 to 10 minutes or until the cheese is melted and lightly browned.

Per serving: Calories: 249; Total Fat: 19g; Total Carbs: 9g; Fiber: 3g; Net Carbs: 6g; Protein: 12g
Macronutrients: Fat: 70%; Protein: 18%; Carbs: 12%

Bacon-Wrapped Asparagus

Serves 6
Prep time: 10 minutes

Cook time: 15 minutes
Total time: 25 minutes

Fresh, crisp asparagus is possibly my favorite vegetable. This recipe uses bacon to hold the asparagus in tasty little bundles. When wrapping, be sure to spread the bacon out evenly across the bundle with little overlap. This ensures the bacon gets crispy while cooking.

2 pounds asparagus spears
2 tablespoons olive oil
½ teaspoon freshly ground black pepper

¼ teaspoon salt
6 bacon slices

1. Preheat the oven to 400°F. Line a baking sheet with a piece of crinkled aluminum foil.

2. Divide the asparagus stalks evenly into 6 bundles.

3. Lightly drizzle the asparagus with the oil, season with the pepper and salt, and toss to coat. Wrap each asparagus bundle with a slice of bacon, using a toothpick to hold it in place.

4. Arrange the bundles on the baking sheet and bake for 12 to 15 minutes or until the bacon is crisp.

5. Remove the toothpicks and serve.

METHOD TIP: This recipe also works great on the grill. Follow the steps as written, then, instead of cooking on a baking sheet, place the bundles on the grill over indirect heat for about 12 minutes or until the bacon is crisp.

Per serving: Calories: 124; Total Fat: 9g; Total Carbs: 6g; Fiber: 3g; Net Carbs: 3g; Protein: 7g
Macronutrients: Fat: 63%; Protein: 20%; Carbs: 17%

Roasted Green Bean Almandine with Blistered Tomatoes

Serves 6
Prep time: 5 minutes

Cook time: 15 minutes
Total time: 20 minutes

Almandine (or almondine or amandine, depending on where you live) simply means a dish baked in butter and seasonings and garnished with flaked almonds. Years ago, I worked at a small seafood restaurant that would "almandine" almost anything: red snapper, scallops, green beans, and a dozen other items. Those dishes were wildly popular because they were so delicious. The crispy, slivered almonds (available in the bulk section of the grocery store for a fraction of the cost of prepackaged options) are the perfect complement to fresh fish and vegetables. Enjoy my take on one of the restaurant's most popular side dishes.

1½ pounds green beans
6 large cherry tomatoes, halved
3 tablespoons melted butter
1 teaspoon garlic powder
½ teaspoon onion powder

½ teaspoon salt
½ teaspoon freshly ground black pepper
½ cup slivered almonds
Juice of 1 lemon (2 tablespoons)

1. Preheat the oven to 450°F.

2. Spread the green beans and tomatoes on a baking sheet in a single layer. Drizzle with the melted butter. Season with the garlic powder, onion powder, salt, and pepper. Toss to coat.

3. Bake for 15 minutes or until the green beans are softened and have browned spots.

4. Transfer to a serving platter, sprinkle with the slivered almonds, and squeeze the lemon juice over the top. Serve.

Per serving: Calories: 145; Total Fat: 11g; Total Carbs: 11g; Fiber: 5g; Net Carbs: 6g; Protein: 4g
Macronutrients: Fat: 62%; Protein: 9%; Carbs: 29%

Loaded Mashed Cauliflower

Serves 6
Prep time: 10 minutes

Cook time: 10 minutes
Total time: 20 minutes

You don't have to miss out on loaded mashed potatoes just because you're eating keto. This loaded cauliflower is equally comforting and filling. It reheats beautifully for serving during the rest of the week. Just microwave for a few minutes, or better yet, stir in a tablespoon or two of heavy cream and reheat on the stove over medium-low heat. This recipe will quickly become a family favorite. If it does, I strongly suggest purchasing a potato masher. This tool only costs a couple of dollars at most but is incredibly good at turning cauliflower into "mashed potatoes."

---

1 head cauliflower, cut into 1-inch pieces
⅓ cup water
½ teaspoon onion powder
½ teaspoon garlic powder
1 teaspoon salt
½ teaspoon freshly ground black pepper

2 tablespoons butter
¼ cup heavy cream
1½ cups shredded cheddar cheese
3 tablespoons bacon bits or crumbled cooked bacon
2 scallions, sliced (green parts only)

1. Place the cauliflower in a large saucepan with the water. Cover and bring to a boil. Lower the heat to medium-low and cook, covered, for about 10 minutes or until fork-tender. Remove the lid for the last 2 minutes to allow the water to evaporate, stirring frequently. Do not allow the cauliflower to burn.

2. Drain any excess water from the pot. Using a potato masher or large spoon, mash the cauliflower to the consistency of lumpy mashed potatoes.

3. Add the onion powder, garlic powder, salt, pepper, butter, cream, cheese, bacon, and scallions to the pot and stir well to combine and melt the butter and cheese with the residual heat. Serve warm.

Per serving: Calories: 232; Total Fat: 19g; Total Carbs: 6g; Fiber: 2g; Net Carbs: 4g; Protein: 11g
Macronutrients: Fat: 73%; Protein: 17%; Carbs: 10%

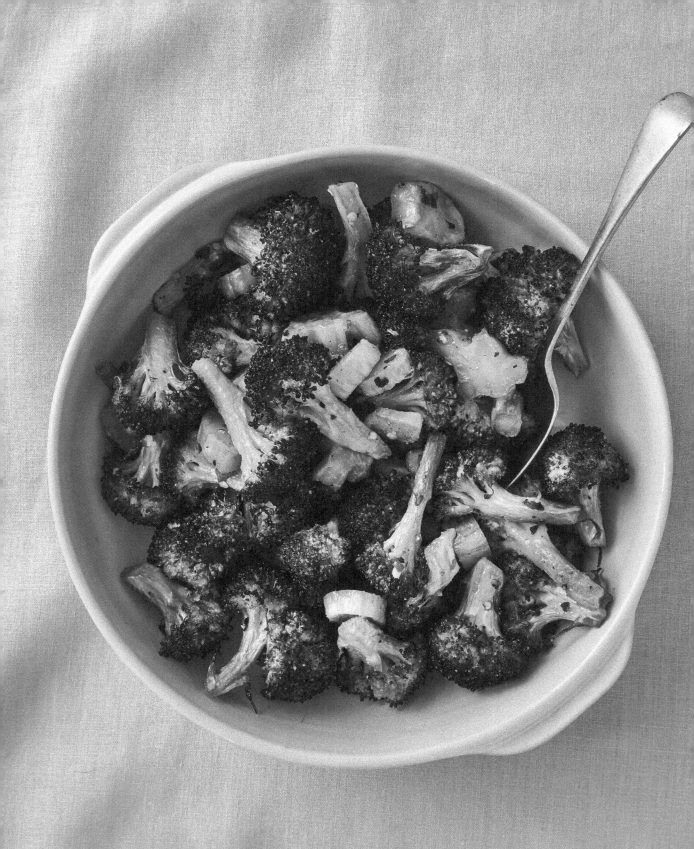

Crispy Pan-Roasted Broccoli

Serves 6
Prep time: 5 minutes

Cook time: 15 minutes
Total time: 20 minutes

For those who've only had steamed broccoli, this recipe will be a revelation. This couldn't be an easier side dish to prepare, and the payoff is huge. The broccoli browns and crisps. This recipe is great made with melted butter, and it's outstanding with melted bacon fat. (If using bacon fat, reduce the added salt by half.) The optional red pepper flakes add a light heat.

Oil, for greasing baking sheet
1 pound fresh broccoli
3 tablespoons melted butter or bacon fat
½ teaspoon onion powder

½ teaspoon garlic powder
1 teaspoon salt
½ teaspoon freshly ground black pepper
½ teaspoon red pepper flakes (optional)

1. Preheat the oven to 425°F. Line a large baking sheet with aluminum foil and lightly oil or spray with cooking spray.

2. Break the broccoli florets into 1- to 2-inch bite-size pieces. Peel off the outer layer of the broccoli stems, trim the end, and chop into 1-inch pieces.

3. Spread out the broccoli on the baking sheet and drizzle with the melted butter. Evenly sprinkle with the onion powder, garlic powder, salt, pepper, and red pepper flakes (if using) and use a spatula to toss to coat. Spread the broccoli out again.

4. Roast on the center oven rack for 12 to 15 minutes or until the broccoli is cooked and lightly browned, tossing halfway through. Serve warm.

Per serving: Calories: 78; Total Fat: 6g; Total Carbs: 5g; Fiber: 2g; Net Carbs: 3g; Protein: 2g
Macronutrients: Fat: 68%; Protein: 7%; Carbs: 25%

Easy Cauliflower Rice

Serves 6 to 8
Prep time: 10 minutes

Cook time: 20 minutes
Total time: 30 minutes

Cauliflower rice is a staple in many keto households. You can purchase frozen riced cauliflower, and although it's useful for a quick meal, this recipe ups the ante and makes a toasty, flavorful rice that far surpasses any frozen product I've tried. Depending on the season, fresh cauliflower may cost less than frozen, providing more servings for the same money. If your head of cauliflower is particularly large, you may need to roast it in two batches. To ensure that it dries out and toasts, rather than becomes soggy, spread the cauliflower into a thin layer.

---

2 teaspoons olive oil, plus more for greasing baking sheet
1 head cauliflower

1 teaspoon salt

1. Preheat the oven to 450°F. Line a baking sheet with aluminum foil and lightly coat with oil or nonstick cooking spray.

2. Using a box grater over a large bowl, grate the entire head of cauliflower, including the stems, into rice-size pieces.

3. Drizzle the oil and salt over the cauliflower rice and stir well to lightly coat.

4. Spread the cauliflower rice evenly on the pan and roast on the center oven rack for 10 minutes.

5. Remove from the oven and use a spatula to toss the rice. Spread it back out and roast for another 10 minutes.

6. Repeat step 5, roasting in 5-minute increments until the cauliflower rice is lightly toasted and done.

7. Serve immediately with your favorite sauce or entrée.

8. Store leftovers in an airtight container in the refrigerator for up to 5 days, or portion and freeze for up to 3 months.

> METHOD TIP: If you have a food processor, you can make quick work of ricing the cauliflower. Cut the head into golf ball–size pieces, then pulse in the food processor in small batches until rice size. Continue with the recipe as written.

Per serving: Calories: 38; Total Fat: 2g; Total Carbs: 5g; Fiber: 2g; Net Carbs: 3g; Protein: 2g
Macronutrients: Fat: 41%; Protein: 12%; Carbs: 47%

Zucchini Noodles

Serves 2
Prep time: 5 minutes

Cook time: 5 minutes
Total time: 10 minutes

Zucchini noodles, or "zoodles," are a popular keto pasta alternative that are delicious with any traditional pasta sauce. Don't overcook these delicate noodles, because they get soft quickly. You'll notice this recipe breaks my initial rule that all recipes in this book would serve 6 to 8 people. That's because these noodles are quick to make and don't reheat very well. It's easy to adjust for extra people by following this simple rule: one medium zucchini per person. Need seven servings? Use seven medium zucchini. Summertime is perfect for buying large batches of ripe zucchini at very low prices. They last 5 to 7 days in the refrigerator.

2 medium zucchini
1 teaspoon olive oil

½ teaspoon salt
½ teaspoon freshly ground black pepper

1. Trim the ends of the zucchini. Using a sharp vegetable peeler, carefully slice off thin, noodle-size pieces by gliding the peeler along the zucchini from end to end. (This is easier to do by resting the zucchini on a cutting board instead of holding it in your hand.)

2. In a large skillet over medium-high heat, combine the oil, zucchini noodles, salt, and pepper, and gently sauté for about 5 minutes or until the zucchini noodles just become tender. Do not overcook.

3. Serve warm as a side dish or topped with your favorite sauce.

METHOD TIP: If you enjoy zucchini noodles enough that you want to splurge on a device designed specifically for this task, I encourage you to read reviews of both tabletop and handheld "spiralizer" units and purchase one online, where prices are generally lower. There are nice options in both categories.

Per serving: Calories: 53; Total Fat: 3g; Total Carbs: 6g; Fiber: 2g; Net Carbs: 4g; Protein: 2g
Macronutrients: Fat: 48%; Protein: 11%; Carbs: 41%

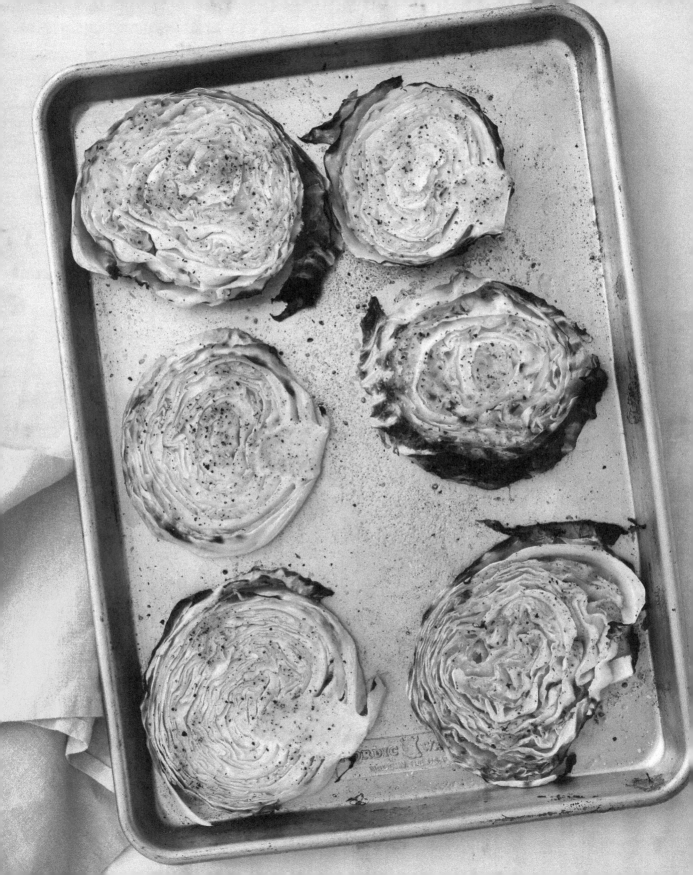

Roasted Cabbage Steaks

Serves 6
Prep time: 5 minutes

Cook time: 20 minutes
Total time: 25 minutes

Cabbage "steaks?" You bet! These delicious, caramelized cabbage rounds are extremely fast and easy to make. As in the Cheesy Sausage and Cabbage Hash recipe (page 25), you can use either red or green cabbage. Both are delicious, but I usually select red for all the heart-healthy anthocyanins that make the cabbage red. The outer edges will get very dark and crispy. (My favorite part.) Enjoy these with your favorite meat or poultry dish; they're perfect alongside an actual steak.

---

1 head red or green cabbage
2 tablespoons olive oil or melted bacon fat
1 teaspoon salt

½ teaspoon freshly ground black pepper
½ teaspoon garlic powder
½ teaspoon onion powder

1. Preheat the oven to 400°F. Line a large baking sheet with aluminum foil.

2. Remove any loose or dark leaves from the outside of the cabbage, and place the head stem-side down on a cutting board. Use a sharp knife to slice the cabbage lengthwise into 6 even slices, about 1 inch thick.

3. Place the cabbage "steaks" on the baking sheet. Brush or drizzle with the oil.

4. Sprinkle the "steaks" with the salt, pepper, garlic powder, and onion powder.

5. Roast on the center oven rack for 15 to 20 minutes or until caramelized. Serve warm.

Per serving: Calories: 85; Total Fat: 5g; Total Carbs: 11g; Fiber: 3g; Net Carbs: 8g; Protein: 2g
Macronutrients: Fat: 50%; Protein: 6%; Carbs: 44%

Pan-Roasted Red Radish "Potatoes"

Serves 6   **Cook time:** 30 minutes
Prep time: 10 minutes   **Total time:** 40 minutes

Roasted radishes are a delicious alternative to roasted red-skinned potatoes. I'm not particularly fond of raw radishes—the sharp, peppery flavor is not something I really enjoy—but the moment you roast or boil them, radishes turn into warm, mild root vegetables that could almost be mistaken for potatoes, in both texture and flavor. I recommend using bacon fat in this recipe for maximum flavor, but olive oil or even melted butter are good options. Enjoy these "potatoes" with any meat recipe, like the Pan-Seared Hanger Steak with Easy Herb Cream Sauce (page 83).

---

2 pounds red radishes, trimmed and halved   ½ teaspoon garlic powder
2 tablespoons melted bacon fat or olive oil   ½ teaspoon onion powder
1 teaspoon salt   ½ teaspoon red pepper flakes (optional)
½ teaspoon freshly ground black pepper   ½ teaspoon Italian seasoning (optional)

1. Preheat the oven to 400°F. Line a large baking sheet with aluminum foil.

2. Spread out the radishes on the baking sheet. Drizzle with the bacon fat. Sprinkle with the salt, pepper, garlic powder, and onion powder, and the red pepper flakes and Italian seasoning (if using) and toss well to coat. Spread out in a single layer.

3. Bake on the center oven rack for 30 to 40 minutes (depending on the size of the radishes) or until golden brown and crispy. Toss halfway through cooking. When done, a fork should pierce the radishes easily.

SUBSTITUTION TIP: If you ever see daikon radishes in your store and they're reasonably priced, pick some up. These long, bright white radishes have a very mild flavor, and when sliced thickly and roasted, they're a convincing potato alternative. Think of them as an option for the red radishes in this recipe.

Per serving: Calories: 64; Total Fat: 5g; Total Carbs: 5g; Fiber: 2g; Net Carbs: 3g; Protein: 1g
Macronutrients: Fat: 64%; Protein: 6%; Carbs: 30%

Creamed Spinach

Serves 6
Prep time: 5 minutes

Cook time: 15 minutes
Total time: 20 minutes

Creamed spinach is a steakhouse classic for a reason: the salty, creamy flavors and texture are irresistible. This recipe replicates the restaurant favorite without the boiling and blanching that is usually called for. You'll need a very large skillet or pot to make this, but the spinach quickly wilts down to a manageable size. You're left with a creamy and cheesy side dish you'll love, with less work than you expected.

3 tablespoons butter
½ medium white onion, diced
2 garlic cloves, minced
½ cup heavy cream
¼ cup water

4 ounces cream cheese, cubed, at room
   temperature
2 pounds bagged baby spinach
⅓ cup shredded Parmesan cheese
1 teaspoon salt
1 teaspoon freshly ground black pepper

1. In a large skillet over medium heat, melt the butter.

2. Add the onion and sauté for 6 to 8 minutes until translucent. Add the garlic and sauté until fragrant, about 1 minute.

3. Add the cream, water, and cream cheese. Stir while melting the cream cheese, 2 to 4 minutes.

4. Stir in half of the spinach. Cook for 2 to 4 minutes until the spinach is wilted. Stir in the remaining spinach and cook until all the spinach is wilted and combined into the cream, 2 to 4 minutes.

5. Remove from the heat and add the Parmesan, salt, and pepper, and stir to combine. Cover and allow to sit for 5 minutes. Stir and serve.

INGREDIENT TIP: If you can't find baby spinach, you can use full-grown spinach. Just massage the leaves in your hands to break up their rough texture before you sauté them.

Per serving: Calories: 247; Total Fat: 22g; Total Carbs: 9g; Fiber: 4g; Net Carbs: 5g; Protein: 8g
Macronutrients: Fat: 77%; Protein: 10%; Carbs: 13%

Southern-Style Collard Greens

Serves 6 to 8
Prep time: 10 minutes

Cook time: 2 hours
Total time: 2 hours 10 minutes

As a true Southerner, nothing says home to me like a big pot of collard greens on the stove. This recipe is easy to make; it just takes some time on the stove to get the consistency right. I often use trimmed and washed collard greens from a bag, but it's much cheaper to buy fresh greens and prepare them yourself. It's going to look like a lot of greens, but they wilt down very quickly. Smoked ham hocks are very affordable and add a tremendous amount of flavor. (The bits of meat are my favorite part.) Look for them at the butcher counter.

2 tablespoons bacon fat or olive oil
2 smoked ham hocks (about ½ pound)
1 medium white onion, diced
3 garlic cloves, minced
4 cups chicken stock
1 cup water

1 teaspoon salt
1 teaspoon freshly ground black pepper
1 teaspoon red pepper flakes (optional)
3 pounds collard greens, stemmed
  and chopped

1. Melt the bacon fat in a large pot over medium-high heat.

2. Add the ham hocks and cook until browned on all sides, about 5 minutes.

3. Add the onion and garlic, and cook until the onion is translucent, about 5 minutes. Stir constantly to prevent the garlic from burning.

4. Add the stock, water, salt, pepper, and red pepper flakes (if using). Cover the pot with a lid. Lower the heat to medium and cook, covered, for 1 hour.

5. Remove the meat from the pot and set aside to cool. When cool enough to touch, use your hands or two forks to pull the meat from the bones and shred into bite-size pieces. Return the meat and stripped bones to the pot.

6. Add the collard greens. Cover the pot and cook on medium heat for at least 1 hour or until tender and done.

7. Remove the bones from the pot. Stir and serve.

SUBSTITUTION TIP: If you can't find ham hocks, a turkey neck or even a turkey leg works well, too. Just follow the recipe as written. This recipe is also great with any tough greens such as mustard greens, kale, or a combination of those.

Per serving: Calories: 195; Total Fat: 9g; Total Carbs: 21g; Fiber: 10g; Net Carbs: 11g; Protein: 13g
Macronutrients: Fat: 39%; Protein: 21%; Carbs: 40%

Crispy Pan-Roasted Okra

Serves 6
Prep time: 5 minutes

Cook time: 15 minutes
Total time: 20 minutes

Many people who have had bad experiences with okra might think of it as slimy, mushy, and usually boiled. Although that is certainly the way many people enjoy eating it, okra takes on a new life when roasted until browned and crispy. Rethink your relationship with this vegetable and try this recipe. It never disappoints, and I've turned die-hard "anti-okra" friends into okra lovers with this simple technique.

1½ pounds whole okra
2 tablespoons olive oil
½ teaspoon salt

½ teaspoon freshly ground black pepper
½ teaspoon dried oregano

1. Preheat the oven to 450°F. Line a large baking sheet with aluminum foil.

2. After washing the okra, let it dry well on a paper towel. Moisture will prevent it from getting crispy and browned.

3. Trim the stem end and the bottom tip off each piece of okra. Place in a large bowl.

4. Drizzle the okra with the oil and season with the salt, pepper, and oregano. Toss to coat evenly.

5. Using your hands, transfer the okra to the baking sheet, leaving any excess oil in the bowl.

6. Roast on the center oven rack for 15 to 20 minutes (depending on the size of the okra) or until the okra is crispy and browned, tossing halfway through cooking. Serve while hot and crisp.

INGREDIENT TIP: The smaller the okra, the more tender it will be. If using larger, older okra, slice them in half lengthwise and continue with the recipe as written.

Per serving: Calories: 77; Total Fat: 5g; Total Carbs: 8g; Fiber: 4g; Net Carbs: 4g; Protein: 2g
Macronutrients: Fat: 54%; Protein: 7%; Carbs: 39%

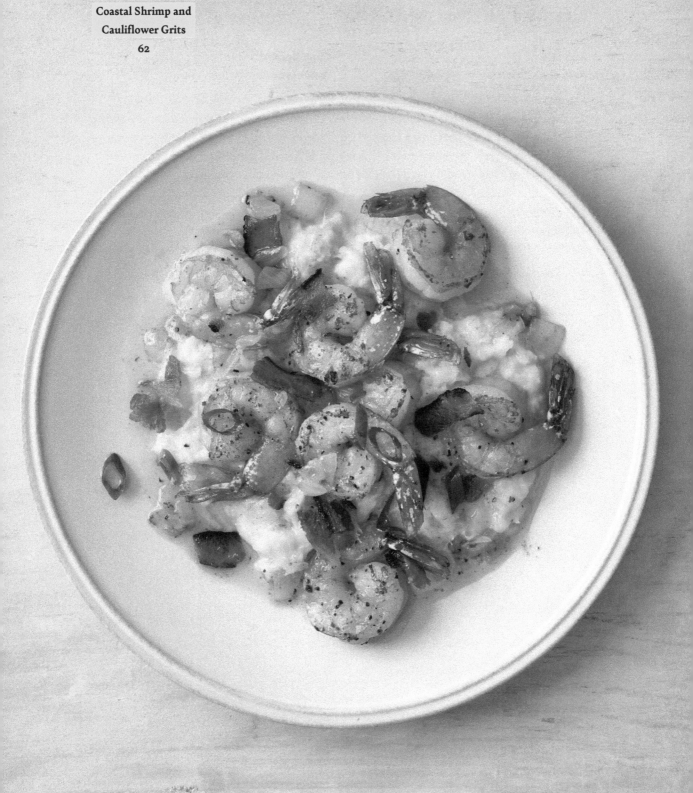

CHAPTER 5

Poultry and Seafood

Coastal Shrimp and
Cauliflower Grits 62

Salmon Croquettes 65

Chicken Divan Casserole 66

Buffalo Chicken Spaghetti
Squash 68

Panfried Tilapia 70

Crispy Chicken Tenders 71

Coconut Chicken Adobo 72

Garlic Parmesan Chicken
Wings 73

Baked Lemon Garlic
Chicken 75

Easy Chicken Alfredo 76

Chicken and Sausage
Jambalaya 77

Sweet and Spicy Turkey
Meatballs 78

Coastal Shrimp and Cauliflower Grits

Serves 6
Prep time: 10 minutes

Cook time: 20 minutes
Total time: 30 minutes

This is perhaps my favorite recipe in this entire book and one of the most popular recipes on my YouTube channel. Shrimp and grits is a Southern coastal staple. Every seafood restaurant from New Orleans to Charleston has a recipe, and it's often the best item on the menu. I eliminated the carb-heavy corn grits and replaced them with a delicious cauliflower alternative. Splurge on a small block of smoked Gouda cheese for best results. Large or jumbo shrimp are ideal here, but medium shrimp will work.

FOR THE GRITS

1 pound frozen cauliflower florets
1 tablespoon butter
3 tablespoons heavy cream
4 ounces smoked Gouda cheese, shredded
Salt
Freshly ground black pepper

FOR THE SHRIMP

6 bacon slices, cut into ½-inch pieces
2 tablespoons butter
⅓ medium white onion, diced
3 garlic cloves, minced
2 pounds shrimp, peeled and deveined
2 to 3 scallions, sliced (green parts only)
Squeeze of lemon juice

TO MAKE THE GRITS

1. In a 9-by-9-inch casserole dish or covered glass bowl, microwave the cauliflower for 10 to 12 minutes, stirring occasionally. Mash with a potato masher or wooden spoon until it becomes thick and granular yet smooth, like the consistency of grits.

2. To the cauliflower, add the butter, cream, and smoked Gouda. Mix well and season with salt and pepper to taste. Keep warm.

TO MAKE THE SHRIMP

3. In a large skillet over medium heat, cook the bacon until crispy. Use a fork or slotted spoon to transfer the bacon to a paper towel.

4. To the remaining bacon fat, add the butter and onion, and cook until lightly browned. Add the garlic and stir until fragrant, about 30 seconds.

5. Add the shrimp. Cook for 8 to 10 minutes or until just cooked and still tender. Remove from the heat and mix in the reserved bacon. Toss to combine.

6. Divide the cauliflower grits between 6 bowls and top generously with the shrimp and sauce.

7. Garnish with the scallions and a squeeze of lemon, and serve.

INGREDIENT TIP: Fresh shrimp are always best, but in the absence of affordable fresh seafood, look for peeled and deveined shrimp in the frozen section. Be sure to select raw shrimp and not precooked shrimp. Thaw the raw shrimp in a colander under cool running water and pat dry with a paper towel before proceeding with the recipe.

Per serving: Calories: 343; Total Fat: 18g; Total Carbs: 6g; Fiber: 2g; Net Carbs: 4g; Protein: 40g
Macronutrients: Fat: 47%; Protein: 47%; Carbs: 6%

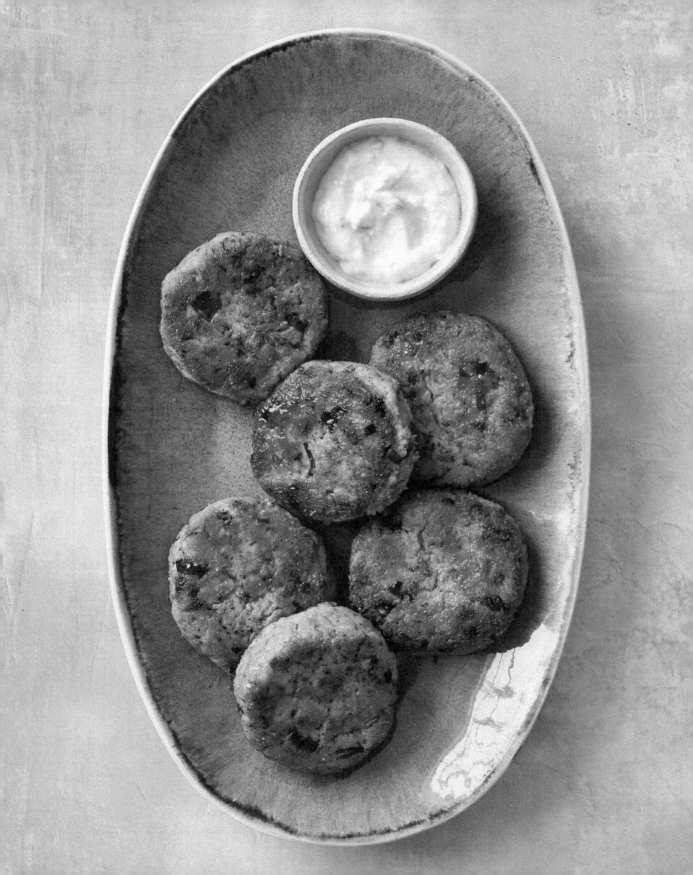

Salmon Croquettes

Makes 6
Prep time: 5 minutes, plus 30 minutes for chilling

Cook time: 15 minutes
Total time: 50 minutes

Growing up, these were a quick Sunday-night supper that the whole family loved. These crispy little fish patties are great served alongside mashed potatoes or cheese grits, so they work perfectly using the grits from the Coastal Shrimp and Cauliflower Grits recipe (page 62). Old Bay Seasoning really makes these croquettes shine. It's a hard seasoning to replicate, but it isn't an absolute necessity. If you do have it, definitely use it.

1 (14.75-ounce) can pink or red
  salmon, drained
½ cup almond flour
1 egg, beaten
1 tablespoon mayonnaise
1 tablespoon lemon juice
2 or 3 scallions, sliced

¼ cup finely minced celery or red
  bell pepper
½ teaspoon dried dill
¼ teaspoon freshly ground black pepper
¼ teaspoon Cajun seasoning
¼ teaspoon Old Bay Seasoning (optional)
Olive oil or butter, for frying

1. In a large bowl, combine the salmon, flour, egg, mayonnaise, lemon juice, scallions, celery, dill, pepper, Cajun seasoning, and Old Bay Seasoning (if using) and mix well.

2. Using your hands, form the mixture into 6 patties about 1 inch thick. Refrigerate the patties for 30 minutes.

3. Heat a thin layer of oil in a skillet over medium heat and fry the patties for 3 to 4 minutes per side, using a spatula to turn.

4. When golden brown, transfer the croquettes to a paper towel–lined plate or onto a baking rack over a baking sheet.

5. Serve with a hearty side dish and your favorite condiment (tartar sauce, remoulade, or even sugar-free ketchup).

SUBSTITUTION TIP: These croquettes can be made with any canned seafood. Try this recipe with a couple small cans of salad shrimp or crabmeat for delicious shrimp cakes and crab cakes. It also works with canned tuna.

Per serving: Calories: 185; Total Fat: 13g; Total Carbs: 2g; Fiber: 1g; Net Carbs: 1g; Protein: 16g
Macronutrients: Fat: 62%; Protein: 34%; Carbs: 4%

Chicken Divan Casserole

Serves 6　　　　　　　　　　**Cook time:** 25 minutes
Prep time: 25 minutes　　　　**Total time:** 50 minutes

This classic dish, which is named after an old French restaurant in New York City, originally featured a béchamel sauce of flour, cream, and butter. Chicken Divan found a second life with home cooks in the 1960s and '70s, who made it with condensed cream of chicken soup. Because neither of those sauces are an option on the keto diet, I've created a version using a quick cream sauce made with sautéed mushrooms and onions for an authentic taste without all the carbs. Don't let the ingredient list scare you: This dish comes together easily, and the result will have your family requesting it in regular rotation.

---

2 tablespoons butter, plus more for greasing the dish
1 tablespoon bacon fat or olive oil
1½ pounds boneless, skinless chicken thighs, cut into 1-inch pieces
1 pound fresh broccoli florets or 1-pound bag frozen
⅓ cup minced white onion
8 ounces white button mushrooms, minced
¾ cup heavy cream

1¼ cups chicken broth
2 ounces cream cheese
½ cup shredded cheddar cheese
⅓ cup mayonnaise
1 tablespoon lemon juice
Salt
Freshly ground black pepper
1 teaspoon curry powder (optional)
½ cup grated Parmesan cheese
¾ cup crushed pork rinds

1. Preheat the oven to 350°F. Butter a 9-by-13-inch casserole dish.

2. Heat the bacon fat in a pan over medium-high heat and brown the chicken until cooked through, 8 to 10 minutes. Remove the chicken and set aside.

3. While the chicken is cooking, steam the broccoli in the microwave until cooked through, 5 to 6 minutes. Drain it well. (This is even easier if you use frozen steam-in-bag broccoli.)

4. Add the butter to the remaining fat in the pan and sauté the onion and mushrooms over medium heat until browned and soft, 8 to 10 minutes.

5. Add the cream, broth, and cream cheese and simmer over medium-low heat for 5 to 7 minutes to reduce, stirring occasionally.

6. Remove the pan from the heat, and stir in the cheddar, mayonnaise, lemon juice, salt, pepper, and curry powder (if using).

7. Spread the cooked chicken and broccoli in the casserole dish, pour the sauce over the top, and smooth the top.

8. In a small bowl, mix the Parmesan cheese and pork rinds, then sprinkle on top of the casserole.

9. Bake for 25 to 30 minutes and serve.

Per serving: Calories: 610; Total Fat: 46g; Total Carbs: 11g; Fiber: 3g; Net Carbs: 8mg; Protein: 38g
Macronutrients: Fat: 68%; Protein: 25%; Carbs: 7%

Buffalo Chicken Spaghetti Squash

Serves 6
Prep time: 15 minutes

Cook time: 1 hour
Total time: 1 hour 15 minutes

Creamy, mildly spicy chicken mixed with delicate spaghetti squash strands makes for a fine casserole. The tang of blue cheese crumbles is the perfect garnish. Spaghetti squash is an incredibly versatile replacement for traditional pasta and very afford-able in the summer and fall. It can be intimidating at first to scrape out the seeds and stringy pit, but it gets easier each time. To halve, place the squash on a cutting board, push a large chef's knife into the center, and pull down on the knife to halve it lengthwise. Turn the squash around and repeat in the other direction.

---

1 large spaghetti squash, halved
2 tablespoons olive oil, divided
¾ cup chicken broth
½ teaspoon salt
½ teaspoon freshly ground black pepper
2 pounds boneless, skinless chicken thighs
4 tablespoons melted butter, divided
1 medium red bell pepper, diced

1 cup Buffalo wing sauce (I like Texas Pete®
  Extra Mild Wing Sauce)
3 ounces cream cheese
1½ cups shredded mozzarella
  cheese, divided
4 green onions, thinly sliced
½ cup blue cheese crumbles

1. Preheat the oven to 350°F. Line a baking sheet with parchment or aluminum foil.

2. Use a large spoon to scrape out and discard the seeds and stringy middle portion of each squash half.

3. Brush the cut sides of the squash with olive oil. Place the squash cut-side down on the baking sheet and roast for 45 minutes or until the squash is tender. (Cooking time will depend on the size of the squash. A sharp knife should easily pierce the squash when it's done.) Allow to cool.

4. While the squash is roasting, cook the chicken. In a large skillet over medium-high heat, combine the remaining olive oil, broth, salt, and pepper. Add the chicken. When the broth comes to a boil, lower the heat to medium-low and cover the skillet. Cook for 20 minutes or until the chicken is done.

5. Transfer the chicken to a large mixing bowl. Shred the meat with two forks.

6. Drain the liquid from the warm pan and reserve.

7. Return the pan to medium heat, add 2 tablespoons of melted butter, and sauté the bell pepper for 5 minutes, until soft. Transfer the cooked bell pepper to the bowl with the shredded chicken.

8. Return the pan to medium heat. Add the wing sauce, cream cheese, and remaining 2 tablespoons of butter. Whisk continuously until the butter and cream cheese are melted.

9. Shred the cooled spaghetti squash into loose noodles and add to the bowl with the chicken and bell pepper. Add 1 cup of the shredded mozzarella and the green onions. Toss everything well to combine.

10. Pour into a 9-by-13-inch baking dish. Evenly distribute the remaining ½ cup of mozzarella cheese and blue cheese crumbles on top.

11. Bake for 10 to 12 minutes to heat through and melt the cheese.

Per serving: Calories: 517; Total Fat: 34g; Total Carbs: 13g; Fiber: 3g; Net Carbs: 10mg; Protein: 41g
Macronutrients: Fat: 58%; Protein: 33%; Carbs: 9%

Panfried Tilapia

Serves 6
Prep time: 5 minutes

Cook time: 25 minutes
Total time: 30 minutes

Panfried fish is delicious and very easy to make. Tilapia is one of the most affordable fish at the seafood counter, but with a watchful eye, you can often find halibut, trout, or even mahi-mahi on sale for a similar price. This recipe calls for using oat fiber as the flour replacement for the dredge. Oat fiber is a specialty item but affordable when ordered online. A bag will last quite a while because it is used sparingly. If you can't find oat fiber (**not oat flour**), then coconut flour is an acceptable alternative, although it doesn't get quite as crispy.

---

6 large tilapia fillets (fresh, or thawed
   if frozen)
½ teaspoon salt
½ teaspoon freshly ground black pepper

2 tablespoons olive oil
½ cup oat fiber or coconut flour
3 tablespoons butter
2 garlic cloves, minced

1. Preheat the oven to 250°F or its lowest temperature. Line a baking sheet with paper towels.

2. Season the fillets on both sides with the salt and pepper.

3. In a large skillet over medium-high heat, heat the olive oil.

4. Pour the oat fiber onto a shallow plate. Dredge the fillets in the oat fiber, covering both sides, and shake to remove the excess.

5. Gently add the fillets to the pan, 1 or 2 at a time so they're not crowded. Panfry for 3 to 4 minutes per side or until the fish flakes easily with a fork.

6. Use a spatula to transfer the cooked fish to the baking sheet and place in the oven to keep warm while you fry the remaining fillets.

7. Turn the heat under the skillet to low, wipe out any excess oil, and add the butter and garlic. Stir until the butter is melted and the garlic is fragrant, 1 to 2 minutes.

8. Serve the fish with the garlic butter spooned over the top.

Per serving: Calories: 263; Total Fat: 13g; Total Carbs: 6g; Fiber: 1g; Net Carbs: 5g; Protein: 30g
Macronutrients: Fat: 45%; Protein: 45%; Carbs: 10%

Crispy Chicken Tenders

Serves 6
Prep time: 10 minutes

Cook time: 30 minutes
Total time: 40 minutes

This keto version of chicken tenders replaces the wheat flour coating with two keto-friendly ingredients: crushed pork rinds and Parmesan cheese. For this recipe, powdered Parmesan (in the green can) is the perfect ingredient because it's low in moisture and already in a powdered form like traditional flour.

2 eggs, beaten
2 tablespoons heavy cream
¾ cup oat fiber (optional)
1½ cups crushed pork rinds
⅓ cup powdered Parmesan cheese in a can

1 teaspoon onion powder
1 teaspoon garlic powder
Olive oil, for frying
2 pounds chicken breast, cut into 2-inch tenders

1. Preheat the oven to its lowest possible temperature. Line a baking sheet with paper towels or set a wire cooling rack on the baking sheet.

2. In a shallow bowl, whisk together the eggs and cream.

3. On a large plate, spread the oat fiber (if using).

4. In a pie plate or small pan, combine the pork rinds, Parmesan, onion powder, and garlic powder, and mix well with a fork.

5. In a large skillet, heat 2 to 3 inches of oil over medium-high heat until the oil is about 350°F, 3 to 4 minutes.

6. Pat the chicken dry with paper towels. Place a few chicken strips in the oat fiber (if using) and coat well. Shake off any excess until a thin layer remains.

7. Dip the chicken in the egg wash. Allow excess egg to drip off, then transfer the chicken to the pork rind mixture and coat the entire strip.

8. Carefully place the tenders in the hot oil. Depending on the size of the skillet, fry 4 or 5 tenders at a time for 6 to 8 minutes per side until browned all over and cooked through. Use tongs to transfer the cooked chicken to the baking sheet. Place in the oven to keep warm while you fry the remaining chicken.

9. Serve with your favorite condiments.

INGREDIENT TIP: You can make this recipe without the oat fiber by dipping the dry chicken directly into the egg wash and then into the pork rind mixture.

Per serving: Calories: 327; Total Fat: 15g; Total Carbs: 2g; Fiber: 0g; Net Carbs: 2g; Protein: 46g
Macronutrients: Fat: 41%; Protein: 3%; Carbs: 56%

Coconut Chicken Adobo

Serves 6 to 8 **Cook time:** 50 minutes
Prep time: 10 minutes **Total time:** 1 hour

This recipe is inspired by a dear Filipino friend who makes the most amazing authentic adobo. Soy sauce is an essential ingredient in adobo, but most keto dieters don't consider soy keto friendly. I use Bragg Liquid Aminos or coconut aminos, which contain no soy but have a similar color and flavor. They can usually be found in the "health food" section of the grocery store.

3 pounds bone-in chicken thighs
2 tablespoons olive oil
1 (13.5-ounce) can full-fat coconut milk
½ cup white vinegar
½ cup water
¼ cup liquid aminos or low-sodium soy sauce

2 teaspoons freshly ground black pepper
1 small white onion, sliced
3 garlic cloves, minced
3 bay leaves
2 or 3 scallions, sliced (green parts only)
Lime wedges, for garnish

1. Pat the chicken dry with a paper towel.

2. In a large pot over medium-high heat, heat the oil until shimmering. Add half of the chicken and cook until lightly browned on both sides, 5 to 7 minutes. Transfer to a plate and repeat with the remaining chicken, also removing it to the plate.

3. While the chicken is cooking, in a medium bowl, combine the coconut milk (shake the can vigorously before opening to incorporate the fat), vinegar, water, liquid aminos, and pepper. Whisk to combine.

4. To the oil in the pot, add the onion and garlic. Cook until the garlic is fragrant, about 2 minutes, stirring constantly so it doesn't burn.

5. Return the chicken to the pot and add the bay leaves. Pour the coconut milk mixture over the chicken. When the liquid starts to approach a boil, lower the heat to medium-low, cover, and allow to simmer for 20 minutes.

6. Remove the lid, gently stir, and allow to simmer for 15 minutes more, uncovered, for the sauce to thicken.

7. Transfer the chicken to a serving platter, spoon over some extra sauce, and garnish with the scallions. Squeeze a bit of lime on top just before enjoying.

Per serving: Calories: 600; Total Fat: 50g; Total Carbs: 5g; Fiber: 0g; Net Carbs: 5g; Protein: 34g
Macronutrients: Fat:73 %; Protein: 24%; Carbs: 3%

Garlic Parmesan Chicken Wings

Serves 6
Prep time: 10 minutes

Cook time: 45 minutes
Total time: 55 minutes

I'm not a huge fan of Buffalo wings, but I love garlic Parmesan wings. These are extra crispy because they're baked at high heat with just oil and a little seasoning. The magic happens after they're tossed in buttery, garlicky Parmesan sauce. These will go fast, so be sure to serve yourself first!

Nonstick cooking spray
2 pounds chicken wings
6 tablespoons olive oil
1 teaspoon salt
1 teaspoon garlic powder

8 tablespoons (1 stick) butter, melted
3 garlic cloves, minced
1 cup grated Parmesan cheese
½ teaspoon red pepper flakes

1. Preheat the oven to 400°F. Line a large baking sheet with crumpled aluminum foil or set an oven-safe cooling rack on the baking sheet. Spray with cooking spray.

2. In a large bowl, combine the chicken, oil, salt, and garlic powder. Use your hands or tongs and toss well to coat.

3. Arrange the wings on the baking sheet so they're not touching, and the rack or foil allows air to flow underneath.

4. Bake for about 45 minutes or until the chicken is crispy and lightly browned. Turn the chicken over halfway through cooking.

5. In a large bowl, whisk together the melted butter, garlic, Parmesan, and red pepper flakes.

6. Add the chicken and use tongs to toss the wings and coat them thoroughly.

7. Transfer the wings to a serving platter, drizzle with the remaining sauce, and serve.

METHOD TIP: If you like your wings extra crispy, return them to the baking sheet after coating them in the sauce, and place under the broiler for 2 to 3 minutes before serving.

Per serving: Calories: 724; Total Fat: 60g; Total Carbs: 3g; Fiber: 0g; Net Carbs: 3g; Protein: 43g
Macronutrients: Fat: 75%; Protein: 24%; Carbs: 1%

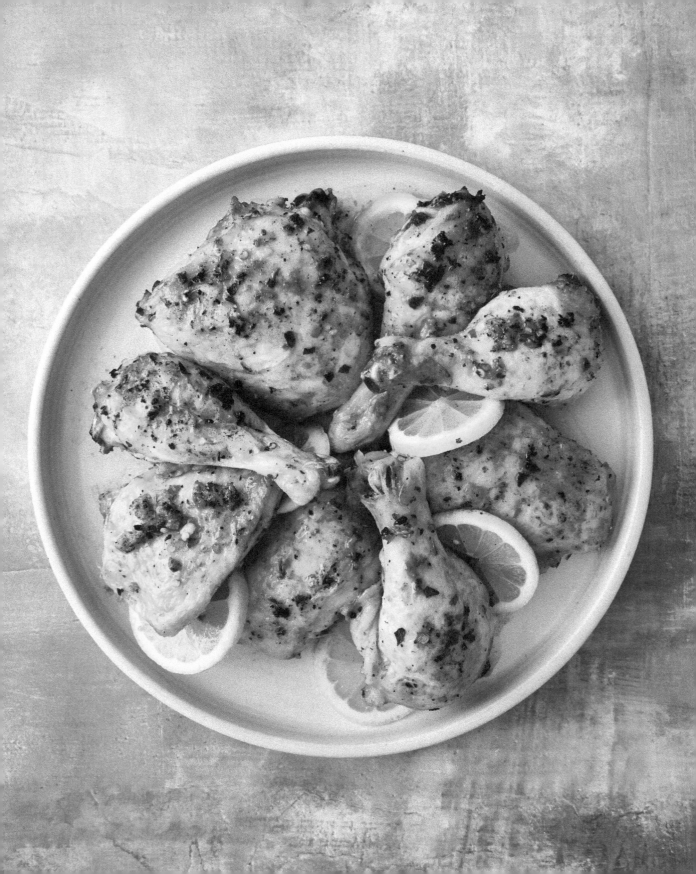

Baked Lemon Garlic Chicken

Serves 6 to 8
Prep time: 10 minutes, plus 30 minutes for marinating

Cook time: 35 minutes
Total time: 1 hour 15 minutes

This family-friendly recipe calls for dark meat leg quarters for moist and juicy chicken, while also hitting those keto fat macros. Marinating the chicken for up to an hour really amps up the flavor, but don't let it marinate any longer than that because the acid in the lemon juice can start to "cook" the chicken. This recipe is delicious served with Crispy Pan-Roasted Okra (page 59). They can cook together at 375°F; just slightly increase the baking time for the okra to compensate for the lower temperature.

---

4 tablespoons olive oil
4 tablespoons lemon juice
4 garlic cloves, minced
1 teaspoon salt

1 teaspoon freshly ground black pepper
½ teaspoon red pepper flakes
4 chicken leg quarters, skin-on, separated
1 lemon, sliced, for serving

1. In a large bowl, whisk together the oil, lemon juice, garlic, salt, pepper, and red pepper flakes.

2. Add the chicken to the marinade and toss well to coat. Cover with plastic wrap and refrigerate for at least 30 minutes and up to 1 hour. Toss halfway through marinating.

3. Preheat the oven to 375°F. Line a large baking sheet with aluminum foil.

4. Toss the chicken a third time to coat it well, then arrange on the baking sheet so the pieces are not touching.

5. Spoon about 1 teaspoon of leftover marinade over the top of each piece of chicken and discard the rest.

6. Bake for 30 to 35 minutes or until the chicken reaches an internal temperature of 165°F when checked with a meat thermometer.

7. Garnish with the lemon slices and serve.

Per serving: Calories: 576; Total Fat: 46g; Total Carbs: 2g; Fiber: 0g; Net Carbs: 2g; Protein: 38g
Macronutrients: Fat: 71%; Protein: 28%; Carbs: 1%

Easy Chicken Alfredo

Serves 6
Prep time: 5 minutes

Cook time: 15 minutes
Total time: 20 minutes

I love to serve this no-fuss chicken and Alfredo sauce over sautéed, sliced zucchini, Zucchini Noodles (page 53), spaghetti squash, or shirataki noodles. (You can usually find the latter, made from plant fiber, near the tofu in the produce section of your grocery store.) The chicken broth enhances the flavor just perfectly for serving with chicken, and the small amount of cream cheese creates a velvety, creamy texture. This dish can be stored in the refrigerator and slowly reheated on the stove; you may want to add a tablespoon or two of water to loosen it up when reheating.

---

2 tablespoons butter
1½ pounds boneless, skinless chicken
   thighs, cut into 1-inch pieces
3 garlic cloves, minced
⅔ cup chicken broth

1 cup heavy cream
4 ounces cream cheese, cubed
½ teaspoon salt
½ teaspoon freshly ground black pepper
¼ teaspoon ground nutmeg (optional)

1. In a large skillet over medium-high heat, melt the butter and add the chicken. Cook for 10 minutes or until the chicken is fully cooked, stirring frequently for even browning.

2. Remove the chicken from the skillet with a slotted spoon and set aside. Reduce the heat to medium.

3. Add the garlic and cook until fragrant, about 30 seconds.

4. Add the broth and use a wooden spoon to scrape the bottom of the pan to deglaze.

5. Add the cream, cream cheese, salt, pepper, and nutmeg (if using), and stir constantly at the bottom to prevent sticking. Simmer for 5 minutes or until the cream cheese has melted and the sauce has reduced to your desired thickness. If the sauce is too thick, thin with a little more cream or broth.

6. Serve with the chicken pieces on top of spaghetti squash, zucchini noodles, or your favorite pasta replacement.

Per serving: Calories: 385; Total Fat: 30g; Total Carbs: 3g; Fiber: 0g; Net Carbs: 3g; Protein: 25g
Macronutrients: Fat: 70%; Protein: 28%; Carbs: 2%

Chicken and Sausage Jambalaya

Serves 6 to 8
Prep time: 10 minutes

Cook time: 45 minutes
Total time: 55 minutes

Jambalaya is best known as a Louisiana staple, and has West African, French, Spanish, and Native American influences. My keto version takes some liberties to lower the carbs, but the flavors are still there. This keto jambalaya is delicious fresh from the stove and even better the next day.

---

2 tablespoons olive oil or bacon fat
1½ pounds boneless, skinless chicken thighs
½ teaspoon salt
½ teaspoon freshly ground black pepper
12 ounces andouille or kielbasa sausage, cut into 1-inch rounds
2 tablespoons butter
1 small white onion, diced
1 bell pepper, diced

2 celery stalks, sliced
3 garlic cloves, minced
1 jalapeño pepper, seeded and diced (optional)
1 tablespoon Cajun seasoning
2 cups low-sodium chicken broth, divided
2 (10-ounce) bags frozen cauliflower rice, thawed, or 20 ounces Easy Cauliflower Rice (page 52)

1. In a large pot over medium heat, warm the oil until it shimmers.

2. Pat the chicken dry with a paper towel, season with the salt and pepper, and add to the pot. Cook for 12 to 15 minutes or until fully cooked through, turning occasionally. Remove to a cutting board and when cool, shred with two forks.

3. In the remaining fat in the pot, brown the sausage until warmed through, about 5 minutes. Remove from the pot with a slotted spoon and reserve.

4. To the pot, add the butter, onion, bell pepper, celery, garlic, jalapeño, and Cajun seasoning, and cook, still over medium heat, for 8 to 10 minutes or until the vegetables are soft and the onion is translucent.

5. Add 1 cup of broth and scrape the bottom of the pot with a wooden spoon to deglaze.

6. Return the chicken and sausage to the pot. Cook the mixture, stirring, for about 8 minutes or until heated through.

7. Add the cauliflower rice and stir well. Continue to cook for 5 minutes until the cauliflower is soft and the contents of the pot are heated through. Turn off the heat, cover, and allow to sit for 5 minutes. (If it gets too thick, add more broth as needed.) Serve warm.

Per serving: Calories: 464; Total Fat: 31g; Total Carbs: 13g; Fiber: 3g; Net Carbs: 10g; Protein: 33g
Macronutrients: Fat: 60%; Protein: 29%; Carbs: 11%

Sweet and Spicy Turkey Meatballs

Serves 6
Prep time: 15 minutes

Cook time: 20 minutes
Total time: 35 minutes

These irresistible meatballs are great as an appetizer or an entrée served with Easy Cauliflower Rice (page 52) and a big green salad. This recipe calls for liquid aminos instead of soy sauce. This is usually found in the "health food" section of the grocery store and has the same flavor profile as soy sauce but without the soy that makes it keto unfriendly. Be sure that the granulated erythritol sweetener is fully dissolved into the sauce. If you happen to have golden erythritol sweetener, that's even better; it adds a hint of brown sugar flavor.

FOR THE MEATBALLS

2 pounds ground turkey
2 eggs, beaten
⅓ cup almond flour
3 tablespoons liquid aminos
1 jalapeño pepper, seeded, finely minced
¼ cup grated white onion

FOR THE SAUCE

½ cup liquid aminos
4 tablespoons granulated erythritol sweetener
½ teaspoon garlic powder
½ teaspoon onion powder
½ teaspoon ground ginger
½ teaspoon freshly ground black pepper

TO MAKE THE MEATBALLS

1. Preheat the oven to 375°F. Line a large baking sheet with crumpled aluminum foil to allow airflow.

2. In a large bowl, combine the turkey, eggs, almond flour, liquid aminos, jalapeño, and onion. Mix with a large spoon or your hands until just combined. (Overmixing can make the meat tough.)

3. Use a spoon to form about 30 uniform meatballs. Roll them gently between your hands to make a tight ball and arrange them on the baking sheet so they're not touching. (You may need two baking sheets, or you can bake in batches.)

4. Bake for 12 to 15 minutes or until cooked through. Turn the broiler to high, move the baking sheet to the top rack, and broil for 2 minutes to brown.

TO MAKE THE SAUCE

5. While the meatballs are cooking, combine the liquid aminos, sweetener, garlic powder, onion powder, ginger, and pepper in a small saucepan and cook over medium-low heat for 10 to 12 minutes. Stir constantly to thicken the sauce and dissolve the granulated erythritol.

6. Transfer the meatballs to a large bowl and pour the sauce over the top. Use a spoon to gently toss and coat them with sauce.

7. Transfer to a serving platter, spoon any remaining sauce from the bowl on top, and serve.

> SUBSTITUTION TIP: This recipe can easily be made with ground pork, lamb, or beef (or any combination of those) instead of ground turkey.

Per serving: Calories: 289; Total Fat: 15g; Total Carbs: 3g; Fiber: 1g; Net Carbs: 2g; Protein: 35g; Erythritol: 8g
Macronutrients: Fat: 47%; Protein: 49%; Carbs: 4%

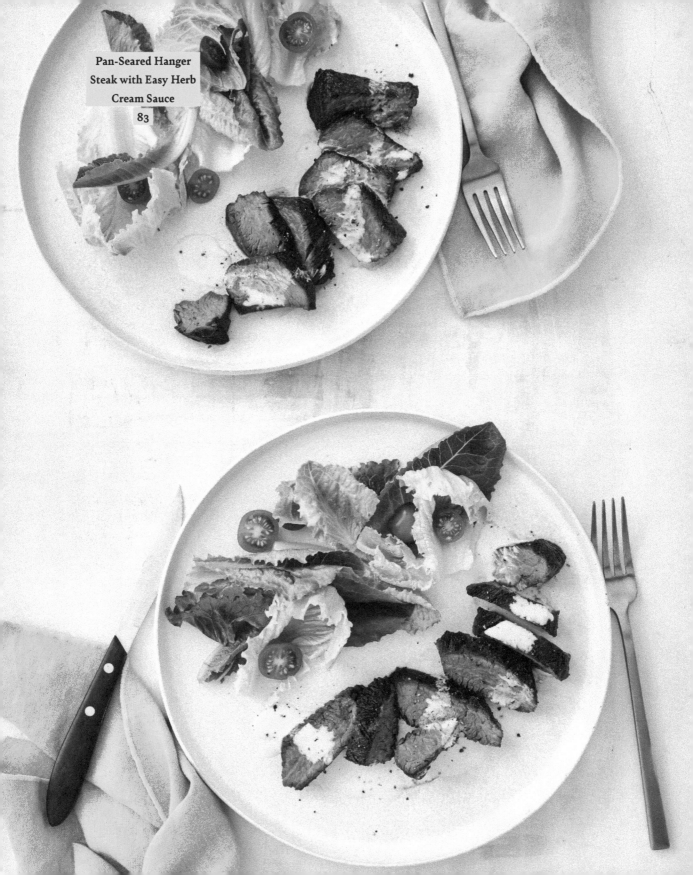

Pan-Seared Hanger
Steak with Easy Herb
Cream Sauce
83

CHAPTER 6

Meat

Easy Mississippi Pot Roast 82

Pan-Seared Hanger Steak with Easy Herb Cream Sauce 83

Cheesesteak-Stuffed Bell Peppers 85

Egg Roll in a Bowl 86

Beef Empanadas 87

Salisbury Steak with Mushroom Gravy 88

Shepherd's Pie 90

Cajun Parmesan Pork Chops 93

Keto Lasagna with Deli Meat "Noodles" 94

Classic Pulled Pork 96

Mom's Pot Roast with Gravy and Radish "Potatoes" 98

Southwest-Style Fajita Bowls 100

Easy Mississippi Pot Roast

Serves 6 to 8
Prep time: 5 minutes
Cook time: 4 to 5 hours on high, 8 to 9 hours on low

Total time: 4 to 5 hours on high, 8 to 9 hours on low

Despite having quite a few pepperoncini peppers, this dish is not spicy at all. The salty vinegar brine helps tenderize the meat (chuck roast is very budget-friendly) and cuts through the rich, fatty gravy made from the meat drippings, butter, and ranch dressing powder. This is best cooked in a slow cooker or low-temperature oven, but see the tip for instructions for making it in a multicooker. Serve with a hearty side dish such as Loaded Mashed Cauliflower (page 49).

---

2 tablespoons olive oil
1 (3- to 4-pound) beef chuck roast
1 packet dry ranch dressing mix

1 (12-ounce) jar pepperoncini
½ medium white onion, sliced
8 tablespoons (1 stick) salted butter

1. Set the slow cooker to high to preheat.

2. Heat a large skillet over high heat, and pour in the oil.

3. Pat the roast with paper towels, then add it to the skillet. Cook for 3 to 4 minutes, browning each side.

4. Place the roast in the slow cooker. Sprinkle the ranch dressing mix over the top.

5. Nestle 8 to 10 whole pepperoncini on and around the roast. Scatter the onion slices over the top. Place the stick of butter on the top center of the roast.

6. Secure the lid on the slow cooker and cook on high for 4 to 5 hours or on low for 8 to 9 hours.

7. When done, remove the whole pepperoncinis and slice them thinly. Reserve.

8. Use two forks to shred the chuck roast. Then return the sliced pepperoncini to the slow cooker and toss to combine.

9. Serve with your favorite hearty side dish.

> METHOD TIP: To make this dish in the oven, use a heavy-duty Dutch oven or a heavy pot with a tight-fitting lid. Cook at 300°F for about 1 hour per pound or until tender when checked with a fork. To cook in a multicooker, combine all the ingredients plus ½ cup of beef broth. Cook on manual high heat for 1 hour, then allow the pressure to naturally release.

Per serving: Calories: 646; Total Fat: 51g; Total Carbs: 3g; Fiber: 1g; Net Carbs: 2g; Protein: 44g
Macronutrients: Fat: 71%; Protein: 27%; Carbs: 2%

Pan-Seared Hanger Steak with Easy Herb Cream Sauce

Serves 4
Prep time: 5 minutes

Cook time: 1 hour
Total time: 1 hour 5 minutes

My friend Misty introduced me to a cream sauce that she serves on just about everything. It's delicious and versatile enough to be used on beef, chicken, pork, vegetables, and even seafood. The hanger steak (sometimes called a "butcher's cut" steak) is a wonderful cut of beef that is affordable and tender.

1 head garlic
1 pint heavy cream
2 to 4 fresh herb sprigs (e.g., tarragon, rosemary)
2 teaspoons salt, divided

1½ pounds hanger steak
1 teaspoon freshly ground black pepper
2 tablespoons olive oil
2 tablespoons unsalted butter

1. Separate the garlic cloves and crush them with a knife. (No need to peel.)

2. In a small saucepan, combine the garlic, cream, herbs, and 1 teaspoon of salt.

3. Simmer, uncovered, on low heat for 1 hour, stirring occasionally. Strain to remove the herbs and garlic.

4. While the sauce is simmering, allow the steak to come to room temperature. Cook the steak when the cream sauce is almost ready.

5. Heat a large, heavy skillet over medium-high heat. Season both sides of the steak with the pepper and the remaining 1 teaspoon of salt.

6. Pour the oil into the hot skillet, then add the steak. Allow it to cook for 4 minutes without lifting or moving it.

7. Turn the steak and add the butter to the pan. Cook the steak for 4 minutes while continuously spooning the melted butter over the top.

8. Transfer to a plate when a thermometer reads 125°F (for medium rare) in the thickest part of the steak. Cover lightly with aluminum foil and allow to rest for 8 to 10 minutes.

9. Thinly slice the steak against the grain. Serve with your favorite side and spoon the cream sauce over the sliced steak.

Per serving: Calories: 884; Total Fat: 80g; Total Carbs: 5g; Fiber: 0g; Net Carbs: 5g; Protein: 37g
Macronutrients: Fat: 81%; Protein: 17%; Carbs: 2%

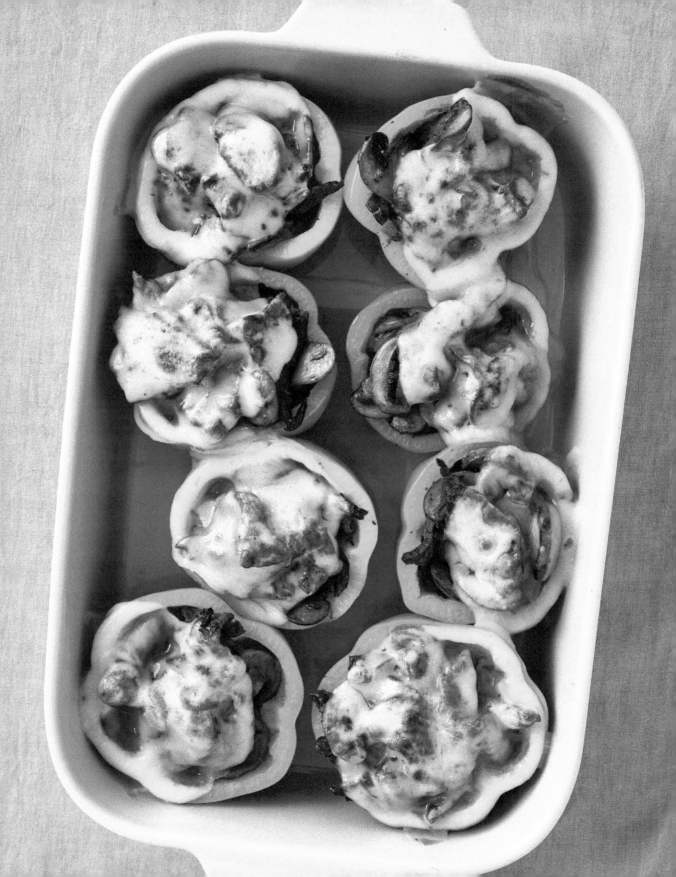

Cheesesteak-Stuffed Bell Peppers

Serves 4 to 6
Prep time: 5 minutes

Cook time: 25 minutes
Total time: 30 minutes

These stuffed bell peppers are a delicious way to satisfy cravings for a giant Philly cheesesteak sandwich without all the carbohydrates of a huge hoagie roll. If you like your cheesesteak sandwiches with a little heat, you can add a minced jalapeño pepper to the onions and mushrooms. Adding some chili powder and cumin to the steak and exchanging the provolone for pepper Jack cheese makes this a delicious Southwest-inspired dish.

4 large bell peppers, halved, seeded, and ribbed
2 tablespoons olive oil
½ medium onion, thinly sliced
12 ounces button mushrooms, sliced
3 garlic cloves, minced

1½ pounds thinly sliced sirloin or shaved beef steak
1 teaspoon salt
1 teaspoon freshly ground black pepper
16 slices provolone cheese

1. Preheat the oven to 350°F.

2. Arrange the bell peppers in a large baking dish, cut-side up, and bake for 15 minutes to soften. Remove from the oven.

3. While the peppers cook, heat a large skillet over medium-high heat. Pour the oil into the hot skillet, then add the onion, mushrooms, and garlic. Sauté until the onion is soft and translucent, about 8 minutes.

4. Add the beef, salt, and pepper. Sauté until the meat is lightly browned, about 8 minutes.

5. Using tongs or a large spoon, evenly distribute the beef mixture between the bell pepper halves.

6. Place 2 slices of provolone cheese on top of each stuffed pepper.

7. Return the peppers to the hot oven for 10 minutes to finish cooking. Turn the broiler on high for the last 2 minutes to lightly brown the cheese. Serve warm.

INGREDIENT TIP: I can usually find prepackaged fresh shaved steak in the meat department. It's typically sold for steak sandwiches. If you can't find that or simply want to splurge a little, select a sirloin steak and ask the butcher to shave it thin enough for sandwiches. They will usually do this at no charge.

Per serving: Calories: 836; Total Fat: 56g; Total Carbs: 17g; Fiber: 5g; Net Carbs: 12g; Protein: 67g
Macronutrients: Fat: 60%; Protein: 33%; Carbs: 7%

Egg Roll in a Bowl

Serves 6
Prep time: 5 minutes

Cook time: 15 minutes
Total time: 20 minutes

This quick dish gives you all the flavors of an egg roll without the pesky non-keto wrapper. You can use a fresh head of cabbage and slice it thin, but for the sake of convenience, I usually pick up a couple of bags of coleslaw mix. It contains a few slivers of carrots, but not enough to throw off the carb count of the final dish. The toasted sesame oil is delicious and really adds to the Chinese-inspired flavor profile, but it's not absolutely necessary. If you happen to have some or want to try it, be sure to add it at the end of cooking and toss well to combine.

2 tablespoons olive oil
2 pounds ground pork
½ small onion, thinly sliced
3 garlic cloves, minced
½ teaspoon salt
½ teaspoon freshly ground black pepper

6 cups coleslaw mix or shredded cabbage
3 or 4 dashes hot sauce
2 teaspoons erythritol sweetener
2 tablespoons liquid aminos or soy sauce
2 teaspoons toasted sesame oil (optional)

1. Heat a large skillet over medium-high heat and pour in the oil.

2. Add the pork, onion, garlic, salt, and pepper. Cook until browned, about 10 minutes.

3. Add the coleslaw mix and toss with the meat.

4. Add the hot sauce, sweetener, and liquid aminos and toss well to coat. Sauté over medium-high heat for 5 to 7 minutes or until the cabbage is wilted and the dish is combined.

5. Remove from the heat and drizzle the sesame oil (if using) over the dish. Toss to combine and serve warm.

SUBSTITUTION TIP: Ground pork is great for this dish, but any ground or minced meat will work, including beef, turkey, and even ground chicken.

Per serving: Calories: 462; Total Fat: 37g; Total Carbs: 5g; Fiber: 2g; Net Carbs: 3g; Protein: 27g; Erythritol: 1g
Macronutrients: Fat: 71%; Protein: 24%; Carbs: 5%

Beef Empanadas

Makes 8
Prep time: 15 minutes

Cook time: 30 minutes
Total time: 45 minutes

Magic Miracle Keto Dough is extremely versatile and really makes these empanadas possible on a keto diet. For most ground-beef dishes, I normally suggest using a high fat ratio, like 80/20, to maintain the fat macros necessary for a keto diet. But using a leaner mixture, like 90/10, in this recipe prevents the beef from making the shell soggy. These freeze well—just let them cool completely first. Reheat in a warm oven to maintain their crispiness.

1 tablespoon olive oil
1 pound lean ground beef
½ cup finely diced white onion
2 garlic cloves, minced
1 teaspoon salt
½ teaspoon freshly ground black pepper

1 teaspoon ground cumin
1 teaspoon paprika
1 batch prepared, uncooked Magic Miracle Keto Dough (page 120)
1 egg, beaten

1. Preheat the oven to 375°F. Line a baking sheet with parchment paper.

2. In a large skillet over medium-high heat, heat the oil.

3. Add the beef, onion, and garlic, and cook until the beef is browned and fully cooked, about 8 minutes. Drain well to remove any excess grease.

4. Add the salt, pepper, cumin, and paprika and cook for 1 to 2 minutes until fragrant. Remove from the heat and allow to cool.

5. Place the prepared dough on 2 pieces of parchment paper. Using a rolling pin, roll out the dough until it is about ¼ inch thick.

6. Use a 6-inch-diameter bowl to cut out 8 circles from the dough. (You may need to gather the dough scraps, knead, and reroll to get all 8 circles.)

7. Spoon a few tablespoons of the meat mixture on half of one dough circle. Fold the other half over and press the edges together firmly to seal.

8. Transfer to the prepared baking sheet. Repeat with the remaining filling and dough circles.

9. Brush the empanadas with the egg. Bake for 15 to 20 minutes or until golden brown. Allow to briefly cool, then serve.

Per serving: Calories: 381; Total Fat: 29g; Total Carbs: 7g; Fiber: 2g; Net Carbs: 5g; Protein: 23g
Macronutrients: Fat: 69%; Protein: 24%; Carbs: 7%

SUPER SAVER

Salisbury Steak with Mushroom Gravy

Serves 6
Prep time: 10 minutes

Cook time: 35 minutes
Total time: 45 minutes

Most kids looked forward to pizza day, but my favorite elementary-school lunch was Salisbury steak and mashed potatoes. I loved that delicious gravy goodness. My keto version brings those flavors and memories to life without the carbs. After browning the steaks, pour off the grease, but be sure to leave any stuck-on browned bits in the pan, because those will help make the gravy brown. If you have room after the gravy is made, put the steaks in the gravy and allow them to sit, covered, for a few minutes to come together. Serve with Loaded Mashed Cauliflower (page 49).

FOR THE STEAKS

2 pounds ground beef
⅓ cup almond flour
¼ cup diced white onion
2 eggs, beaten
¼ cup beef broth
1 tablespoon Worcestershire sauce
1 teaspoon salt
½ teaspoon freshly ground black pepper
½ teaspoon garlic powder
2 tablespoons olive oil

FOR THE GRAVY

3 tablespoons butter
6 ounces button mushrooms, sliced
¼ cup diced white onion
1½ cups beef broth
2 tablespoons Worcestershire sauce
2 ounces cream cheese
¼ cup sour cream
1 teaspoon salt
½ teaspoon freshly ground black pepper
½ teaspoon garlic powder

TO MAKE THE STEAKS

1. In a large mixing bowl, combine the beef, almond flour, onion, eggs, broth, Worcestershire sauce, salt, pepper, and garlic powder. Mix well with your hands to combine.

2. Form into 6 equal patties about 2 inches thick.

3. Heat a large skillet with a lid over medium heat and pour in the oil.

4. Place 3 steaks in the hot oil. Cook, covered, for 5 minutes. Turn the steaks and cook for 5 more minutes. When the steaks are fully cooked, transfer them to a plate and cover with aluminum foil to retain the heat. Cook the second batch.

5. Drain the grease from the skillet but leave behind any stuck-on browned meat.

TO MAKE THE GRAVY

6. Add the butter, mushrooms, and onion to the skillet used to cook the steaks. Sauté for 8 minutes or until the onion is soft and translucent, using a wooden spoon to scrape the browned bits from the bottom of the skillet.

7. Increase the heat to medium-high. Add the broth, Worcestershire sauce, cream cheese, sour cream, salt, pepper, and garlic powder to the skillet and cook, stirring constantly, for about 5 minutes to melt the cream cheese and thicken.

8. Serve the steaks topped with the mushroom gravy.

Per serving: Calories: 616; Total Fat: 50g; Total Carbs: 8g; Fiber: 1g; Net Carbs: 7g; Protein: 33g
Macronutrients: Fat: 73%; Protein: 22%; Carbs: 5%

Shepherd's Pie

Serves 8
Prep time: 10 minutes

Cook time: 45 minutes
Total time: 55 minutes

Shepherd's pie is a comfort food that spans both time and distance. Popular on multiple continents, the layers of minced meat, tender vegetables, and fluffy potato topping are universally loved. This keto version swaps cauliflower for mashed potatoes and tender green beans for the traditional carrots, all on top of a flavorful base of ground beef. Try substituting ground lamb for beef, to get a truly authentic pub-style classic.

FOR THE CAULIFLOWER

1 pound frozen cauliflower florets
4 tablespoons butter
½ teaspoon salt
½ teaspoon freshly ground black pepper
½ teaspoon onion powder
½ teaspoon garlic powder

FOR THE BEEF

2 pounds ground beef
1 small onion, diced

3 garlic cloves, minced
1 tablespoon Worcestershire sauce
½ teaspoon salt
½ teaspoon freshly ground black pepper

FOR THE VEGETABLES

2 tablespoons butter
½ pound green beans, sliced
½ pound white button mushrooms, sliced
½ teaspoon garlic powder
1 cup shredded cheddar cheese

TO MAKE THE CAULIFLOWER

1. In a large, microwave-safe bowl, combine all the ingredients.

2. Cover with a plate and cook in the microwave for 5 minutes on high. Stir well and cook, covered, for another 5 minutes or until tender.

3. Use a potato masher or large slotted spoon to mash the cauliflower to the consistency of mashed potatoes. Set aside. Preheat the oven to 375°F.

TO MAKE THE BEEF

4. In a large skillet over medium-high heat, combine the beef and onion. Cook until the beef is browned and broken apart and the onion is translucent, about 8 minutes. Drain off any excess fat.

5. Add the garlic, Worcestershire sauce, salt, and pepper, and cook until the garlic is fragrant, about 1 minute.

6. Evenly spread the beef in a 9-by-13-inch baking dish.

TO MAKE THE VEGETABLES

7. In the same skillet used to cook the beef, combine the butter, green beans, mushrooms, and garlic powder. Sauté until the beans are tender, about 8 minutes. Spread the bean mixture on top of the ground beef in the casserole dish.

8. Evenly spread the mashed cauliflower on top. Sprinkle with the cheddar.

9. Bake for 20 minutes. Turn the broiler to high and cook for 5 more minutes to melt the cheese and brown the top. Serve.

METHOD TIP: This recipe uses frozen cauliflower, but fresh cauliflower is also great. Regardless of which you select, the cauliflower can also be steamed on the stovetop instead of cooked in the microwave. Add about an inch of water to the pot, cover, and cook on medium-high heat for about 10 minutes or until the cauliflower is fork-tender.

Per serving: Calories: 460; Total Fat: 36g; Total Carbs: 8g; Fiber: 2g; Net Carbs: 6g; Protein: 26g
Macronutrients: Fat: 71%; Protein: 23%; Carbs: 6%

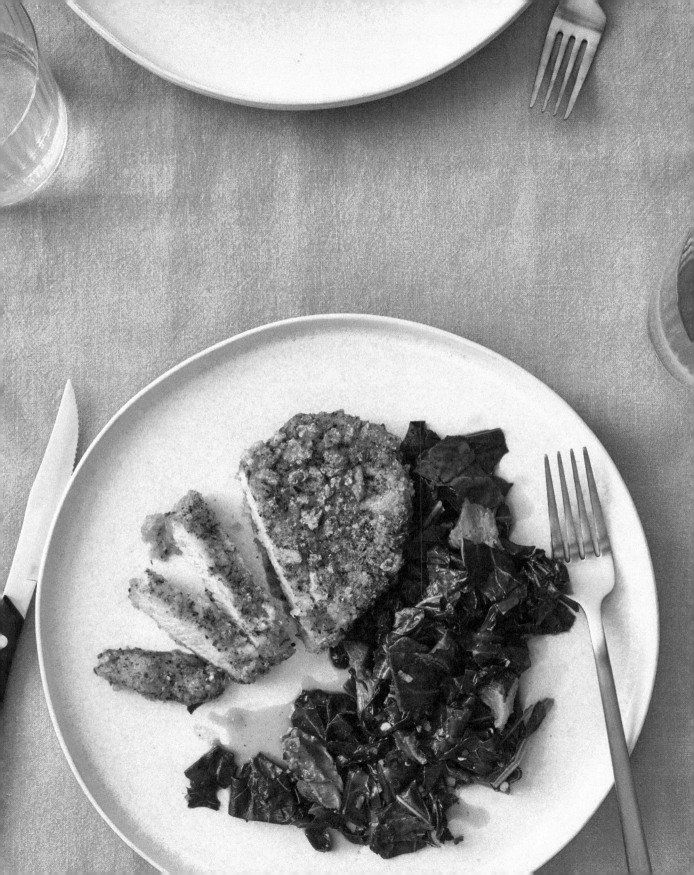

Cajun Parmesan Pork Chops

Serves 6

Prep time: 10 minutes

Cook time: 30 minutes

Total time: 40 minutes

Pork loin chops are often one of the most affordable cuts of meat at the market. You may need to be flexible with the thickness, but there are bargains to be had. Thinner cuts like "breakfast chops" are often on sale; just be mindful to cook them for less time. Likewise, if thick, bone-in pork steaks are on sale, simply increase the cooking time, always aiming for a final temperature of 150°F, regardless of size. These chops are delicious served with Southern-Style Collard Greens (page 58) or Crispy Pan-Roasted Okra (page 59).

Nonstick cooking spray

6 boneless pork loin chops

2 eggs, beaten

2 tablespoons heavy cream

¾ cup oat fiber (optional)

1½ cups crushed pork rinds

⅓ cup powdered Parmesan cheese in a can

2 tablespoons Cajun seasoning

1 teaspoon onion powder

1 teaspoon garlic powder

1. Preheat the oven to 375°F. Line a large baking sheet with crumpled aluminum foil to allow airflow. Spray the foil with cooking spray.

2. Pat the chops dry with a paper towel.

3. In a shallow bowl, whisk together the eggs and heavy cream.

4. Pour the oat fiber (if using) onto a large plate.

5. In a pie plate or small casserole dish, combine the pork rinds, Parmesan, Cajun seasoning, onion powder, and garlic powder, and mix well with a fork.

6. Place a pork chop in the oat fiber and coat it well. Shake off any excess so only a thin layer remains.

7. Transfer the pork chop to the egg wash. Allow excess egg to drip off. Transfer to the pork rind mixture and coat the entire chop. Place the chop on the prepared baking sheet. Repeat with the remaining chops.

8. Bake for 25 to 30 minutes or until the meat registers 150°F at the thickest part of the chop. Allow to rest. Serve with your favorite side dish.

INGREDIENT TIP: Oat fiber is listed as an optional ingredient. You can make this recipe without it by dipping the dry pork chops directly into the egg wash and then into the pork-rind mixture, but the oat fiber really helps the crunchy coating adhere to the chops.

Per serving: Calories: 327; Total Fat: 19g; Total Carbs: 1g; Fiber: 0g; Net Carbs: 1g; Protein: 38g
Macronutrients: Fat: 52%; Protein: 46%; Carbs: 2%

Keto Lasagna with Deli Meat "Noodles"

Serves 8
Prep time: 15 minutes

Cook time: 1 hour 5 minutes
Total time: 1 hour 20 minutes

This lasagna recipe is far from traditional, but the flavors and textures are incredibly close. It has a very unusual ingredient for the "noodles": thinly sliced deli chicken breast. This has become very popular on social media in recent years, with many blogs and websites coming out with their own deli "noodle" lasagna recipes. This is just my standard lasagna recipe but using the clever noodle trick, and it's shocking how much this feels and tastes like "real" lasagna. You'd never know it was chicken! For the sauce, make sure you find a low-carb and sugar-free marinara.

Nonstick cooking spray
1 cup whole-milk ricotta cheese
1 egg
¼ cup shredded Parmesan cheese
3 teaspoons Italian seasoning, divided
½ teaspoon garlic powder
½ teaspoon onion powder
½ teaspoon salt
½ teaspoon freshly ground black pepper

2 tablespoons olive oil
½ medium white onion, diced
3 garlic cloves, minced
2 pounds mild Italian sausage,
   casings removed
2 cups sugar-free marinara sauce
1 pound deli chicken breast, thinly sliced
3 cups shredded mozzarella cheese

1. Preheat the oven to 375°F. Spray a large casserole dish with cooking spray.

2. In a medium bowl, combine the ricotta, egg, Parmesan, 1 teaspoon of Italian seasoning, garlic powder, onion powder, salt, and pepper. Mix well and set aside.

3. In a large skillet over medium heat, heat the oil. Add the onion and sauté until the onion is translucent, about 6 minutes. Add the garlic and remaining 2 teaspoons of Italian seasoning. Cook until fragrant, about 2 minutes.

4. Add the sausage and cook, breaking it up with a spoon, until browned, about 8 minutes.

5. Add the marinara sauce and continue cooking for 10 minutes, uncovered, to thicken. Set aside.

6. Place one-third of the chicken slices in the bottom of the casserole dish. (It helps to cut the round slices in half, so the straight edges fit against the side of the dish.)

7. Use a rubber spatula to spread one-third of the ricotta mixture over the chicken.

8. Spoon one-third of the meat mixture on top of the ricotta and spread evenly.

9. Evenly sprinkle one-third of the mozzarella on top of the meat.

10. Repeat the layers two more times.

11. Bake, uncovered, for about 40 minutes or until the cheese on top is browned and the sides are slightly bubbling.

12. Allow to rest for 10 minutes, divide into 12 slices, and serve with a side salad.

BATCH-COOKING TIP: This recipe is great for batch cooking and meal prep. Once this has cooled completely, refrigerate it in the casserole dish. When chilled, slice it and portion into individual containers that can be refrigerated or frozen and easily reheated.

Per serving: Calories: 708; Total Fat: 55g; Total Carbs: 11g; Fiber: 1g; Net Carbs: 10g; Protein: 42g
Macronutrients: Fat: 70%; Protein: 24%; Carbs: 6%

Classic Pulled Pork

Serves 6 to 8
Prep time: 5 minutes

Cook time: 3 to 4 hours
Total time: 3 to 4 hours

Pork shoulder and pork butt are some of my all-time favorite cuts of meat. (A pork butt isn't really a butt, just a different part of the shoulder.) A low and slow cook allows the collagen to melt away and the meat to become the tender, juicy barbecue goodness we all know and love. I've included instructions for cooking this in the oven, as it requires no special appliances—just a heavy pot or Dutch oven. See the tip for using a multicooker or a slow cooker.

1 tablespoon salt
1 teaspoon freshly ground black pepper
1 teaspoon onion powder
1 teaspoon garlic powder
1 (4- to 5-pound) boneless pork shoulder or pork butt

2 tablespoons olive oil or bacon fat
½ medium white onion, diced
3 garlic cloves, peeled and smashed
12 ounces low-carb beer or low-sodium chicken broth

1. Preheat the oven to 325°F. Arrange the oven racks so the pork will cook in the lower third of the oven.

2. In a small bowl, combine the salt, pepper, onion powder, and garlic powder. Stir to mix well.

3. Cut the pork into baseball-size pieces, and sprinkle with the seasoning mixture, covering all sides.

4. Heat a large Dutch oven or heavy pot with a lid over medium-high heat and pour in the oil.

5. Lightly brown the pork on all sides in batches, 2 to 3 minutes per side.

6. Return all the meat to the pot along with the onion and garlic.

7. Pour the beer over the top so that only a portion of the pork is submerged with some above the liquid.

8. Cover the pot and place it in the oven for 3 to 4 hours. Check for tenderness at about 2 hours, checking every half hour after that. The pork is ready when it is easily shredded with a fork.

9. Transfer the pork to a large bowl or pan. Pour the liquid from the pot into another container, reserving it for use later.

10. Use two forks to shred the meat. Return it to the pot and add as much cooking liquid as needed to moisten. Serve as is or with your favorite low-carb barbecue sauce.

METHOD TIP: To make this dish in a multicooker, season the meat as directed and use the Sauté function to sear the meat in the oil, just until browned on all sides. Press Cancel and pour 8 ounces of beer or broth into the pot, then use a wooden spoon to scrape the bottom to remove any stuck-on bits. Add the onion and garlic and secure the lid. Cook on high pressure for 45 minutes. Allow the pressure to naturally release for 12 minutes, then quick release the remaining pressure and continue with the recipe as written. To make this dish in a slow cooker, follow the recipe as written, but after browning, put the meat in the slow cooker, cover, and cook on high for 4 to 5 hours or on low for 7 to 8 hours.

Per serving: Calories: 632; Total Fat: 42g; Total Carbs: 4g; Fiber: 0g; Net Carbs: 4g; Protein: 54g
Macronutrients: Fat: 61%; Protein: 37%; Carbs: 2%

Mom's Pot Roast with Gravy and Radish "Potatoes"

Serves 8
Prep time: 15 minutes

Cook time: 3 to 4 hours
Total time: 3 to 4 hours

The challenge of making a classic pot roast on a keto diet is finding a thickener for the gravy and a substitute for the potatoes. I've tackled both of those by using red radishes in place of potatoes, and a clever trick of using a few ounces of cream cheese to thicken the gravy. It doesn't taste creamy, but it does give the gravy an unctuous, velvety texture you'd expect from one thickened with flour. This stores very well. Portion the meat into individual storage containers, evenly divide the gravy, cover, and store for up to 5 days in the refrigerator or 3 months in the freezer.

---

1 teaspoon salt
1 teaspoon freshly ground black pepper
1 teaspoon dried thyme
½ teaspoon onion powder
½ teaspoon garlic powder
3 pounds beef chuck roast
2 tablespoons bacon fat or olive oil
1 pound red radishes, trimmed
4 celery stalks, cut into 1-inch slices

1 medium white onion, thickly sliced
3 garlic cloves, sliced
2 bay leaves
1 cup beef broth
¼ cup tomato paste
½ cup red wine or additional beef broth
2 ounces cream cheese, cubed, at room temperature

1. Preheat the oven to 300°F. Arrange the oven racks so the roast will cook in the lower third of the oven.

2. In a small bowl, combine the salt, pepper, thyme, onion powder, and garlic powder and stir to mix well.

3. Pat the roast dry with a paper towel, then season it on all sides with the seasoning mixture.

4. Heat a large Dutch oven or heavy pot with a lid over medium-high heat. Pour in the bacon fat.

5. Brown the roast for 5 minutes on each side. Lower the heat to medium.

6. Arrange the radishes, celery, onion, garlic, and bay leaves around the roast.

7. In a measuring cup, thoroughly whisk the broth and tomato paste together. Pour it over the roast and vegetables. Pour in the red wine.

8. Cover and cook for 3 to 4 hours. Begin checking for tenderness after 2 hours. If the pot is dry, add additional broth to maintain adequate moisture.

9. When the roast is fork-tender, remove it from the oven and allow to rest for 10 minutes.

10. Using a slotted spoon and tongs, transfer the roast and vegetables to a serving platter, leaving the liquid behind.

11. Add the cream cheese to the liquid and whisk well to melt it, allowing it to thicken the gravy. Pour the gravy over the roast and vegetables, and serve.

> **METHOD TIP:** This recipe can be made in a slow cooker. After browning the meat, follow the recipe as written, but reserve the radishes and add them to the slow cooker 2 hours before the end of the cooking time. Cover and cook on high for 4 to 5 hours or on low for 8 to 9 hours. Remove the roast and vegetables from the slow cooker and continue with step 11.

Per serving: Calories: 400; Total Fat: 27g; Total Carbs: 6g; Fiber: 2g; Net Carbs: 4g; Protein: 35g
Macronutrients: Fat: 60%; Protein: 34%; Carbs: 6%

Southwest-Style Fajita Bowls

Serves 6
Prep time: 15 minutes

Cook time: 25 minutes
Total time: 40 minutes

These fajita bowls capture the spirit of Southwest-style, Tex-Mex fajitas without the carbs that come with tortillas. These fajitas are served on a bed of cilantro-lime cauliflower rice for a burst of bright flavor. The ingredient list looks long, but the recipe is quick to put together, and the payoff is worth it. All the ingredients store well in the refrigerator, and it's easy to assemble throughout the week as needed. Reserve half of the marinade to use when assembling the fajitas; it makes a delicious sauce spooned over the cooked steak.

FOR THE MARINADE

1/3 cup olive oil
1/2 cup lime juice
2 garlic cloves, minced
1 teaspoon salt
1 teaspoon chili powder
1/2 teaspoon onion powder
1/2 teaspoon garlic powder
1/2 teaspoon freshly ground black pepper
1/2 teaspoon red pepper flakes
1/2 teaspoon dried oregano
1/2 teaspoon ground cumin
1 or 2 dashes hot sauce (optional)

FOR THE CAULIFLOWER RICE

1 pound frozen riced cauliflower, or Easy
    Cauliflower Rice (page 52)

1 tablespoon olive oil
2 tablespoons lime juice
1/4 cup chopped fresh cilantro (optional)
1 teaspoon salt
1/2 teaspoon ground cumin

FOR THE FAJITAS

2 pounds stir-fry beef or thinly sliced sirloin
3 bell peppers (red or green), sliced
1 medium white onion, halved and sliced

FOR THE GARNISH

Lime wedges
1 avocado, sliced
Sour cream
2 or 3 scallions, sliced

TO MAKE THE MARINADE

1. Combine all the ingredients in a large measuring cup or medium bowl. Reserve half of the marinade.

2. In a large bowl, combine the steak slices and half the marinade. Toss to coat the steak well and allow to sit, covered, for 15 to 20 minutes while you prepare the rice.

TO MAKE THE CAULIFLOWER RICE

3. In a skillet over medium-high heat, sauté the cauliflower in the oil for about 8 minutes or until the cauliflower is the texture of rice.

4. Remove from the heat and add the lime juice, cilantro (if using), salt, and cumin. Mix well. Transfer to a bowl and set aside.

TO MAKE THE FAJITAS

5. Wipe out the skillet and heat it over medium-high heat. When the skillet is hot, put the marinated steak and any marinade left in the bowl into the skillet. Cook, stirring frequently, for 6 to 8 minutes until the steak is cooked through. Transfer to a bowl and set aside.

6. In the same skillet, combine the peppers and onion with 2 tablespoons of reserved marinade. Sauté for about 6 minutes or until the peppers are soft and the onion is translucent.

7. To assemble, divide the cauliflower rice between 6 wide bowls or plates. Top the rice with the steak and vegetables. Spoon a bit of reserved marinade on top. Garnish with lime wedges for squeezing, avocado, a dollop of sour cream, and scallions.

Per serving: Calories: 499; Total Fat: 34g; Total Carbs: 16g; Fiber: 6g; Net Carbs: 10g; Protein: 34g
Macronutrients: Fat: 60%; Protein: 28%; Carbs: 12%

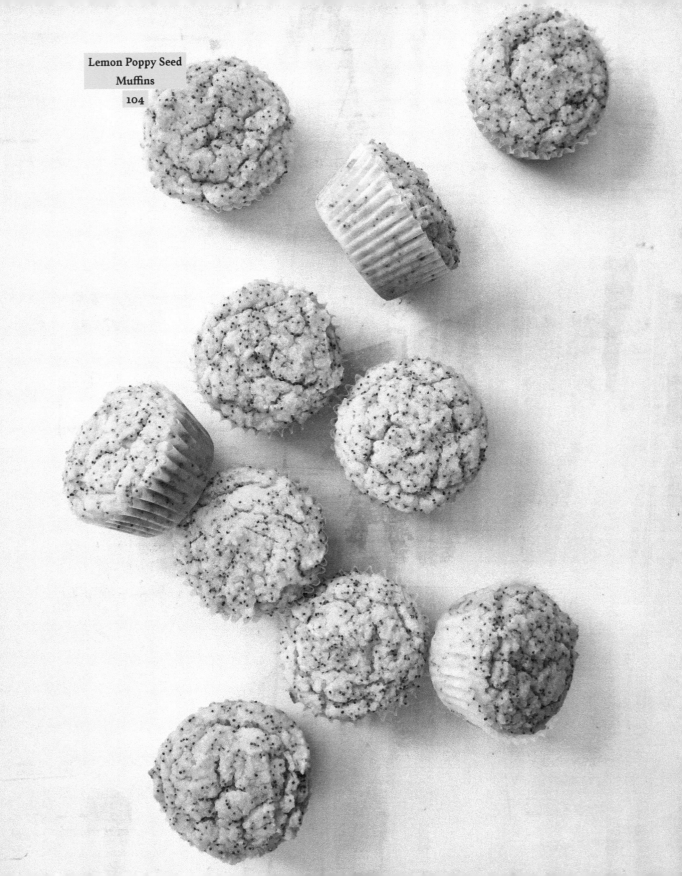

CHAPTER 7

Sweets and Treats

Lemon Poppy Seed
Muffins 104

Quick Pressure Cooker
Cheesecake 105

Old-Fashioned Lemon-Lime
Tea Cakes 106

Summer Squash Mock Apple
Crumble 108

Cinnamon Coffee
Cake 110

Blueberry Cheesecake
Bars 113

Classic Chocolate Chip
Cookies 115

Classic Chocolate
Brownies 117

Lemon Poppy Seed Muffins

Makes 12   **Cook time:** 25 minutes
Prep time: 5 minutes   **Total time:** 30 minutes

These muffins, which were originally developed for my YouTube channel, are great as a fluffy, citrusy breakfast pastry or as a special treat any time of day. One warning: Be sure your poppy seeds are as fresh as possible. Poppy seeds contain enough fat that they can go rancid within a few months of opening, so if you've had a jar of poppy seeds sitting in the pantry for a year or so, toss them out.

¾ cup almond flour
⅓ cup coconut flour
½ cup erythritol sweetener
1 teaspoon baking powder
⅓ cup unsweetened almond milk
¼ cup melted butter

4 eggs
Juice of 1 lemon (2 tablespoons)
Grated zest of 1 lemon (1 heaping tablespoon)
2 tablespoons poppy seeds

1. Preheat the oven to 350°F and place paper liners in the cups of a 12-cup muffin pan.

2. In a large bowl, sift together the almond flour, coconut flour, sweetener, and baking powder.

3. In a separate bowl, whisk together the almond milk, butter, eggs, lemon juice, and lemon zest.

4. Combine the wet and dry ingredients and whisk. Fold in the poppy seeds.

5. Fill the muffin cups evenly.

6. Bake for 20 to 22 minutes until the muffins spring back when touched or a toothpick inserted into a center comes out clean. Allow to cool before serving. Store in an airtight container in the refrigerator with parchment paper between the layers.

SUBSTITUTION TIP: This recipe can easily be altered for blueberry muffins. Omit the poppy seeds and substitute ¼ cup of fresh blueberries.

Per serving: Calories: 104; Total Fat: 8g; Total Carbs: 4g; Fiber: 1g; Net Carbs: 3g; Protein: 4g; Erythritol: 8g
Macronutrients: Fat: 70%; Protein: 15%; Carbs: 15%

Quick Pressure Cooker Cheesecake

Serves 12
Prep time: 5 minutes

Cook time: 30 minutes, plus 3 hours chill time
Total time: 3 hours 35 minutes

This might be the easiest cheesecake recipe ever. The tangy lemon juice and sour cream bring depth of flavor, and the multicooker (I use an Instant Pot) makes quick work of baking a perfect cheesecake. Be sure not to overbeat the mixture when preparing it. This can create a lot of air in the batter, which can cause cheesecakes to crack and fall.

16 ounces full-fat cream cheese, at room temperature
¼ cup sour cream
⅔ cup powdered erythritol

2 eggs, at room temperature
2 teaspoons lemon juice
2 teaspoons vanilla extract

1. In a large bowl, combine the cream cheese, sour cream, and erythritol. Use a hand mixer to beat them until combined.

2. Add the eggs, one at a time, mixing after each addition. Add the lemon juice and vanilla, and mix. Do not overbeat.

3. Butter the inside of a springform pan that fits inside your multicooker. Cover the outside of the pan with aluminum foil to prevent water from entering the springform pan.

4. Pour the cheesecake mixture into the pan.

5. Place the trivet in the bottom of the multicooker and add 1 inch of water. Lower the springform pan onto the trivet.

6. Use the manual setting on high pressure and cook for 20 minutes. Allow a 10-minute natural release, then manually release any remaining pressure.

7. Allow the cake to cool in the multicooker for about 10 minutes, then transfer to a rack for another 10 minutes. Chill for at least 3 hours (preferably overnight for the creamiest texture).

Per serving: Calories: 153; Total Fat: 15g; Total Carbs: 2g; Fiber: 0g; Net Carbs: 2g; Protein: 3g; Erythritol: 11g
Macronutrients: Fat: 86%; Protein: 10%; Carbs: 4%

Old-Fashioned Lemon-Lime Tea Cakes

Makes 20
Prep time: 20 minutes

Cook time: 15 minutes
Total time: 35 minutes

I have a beloved family cookbook that was put together when I was a child. It contains the favorite recipes from all the members of my immediate and extended family. One recipe that caught my eye and brings back memories is my great-grandmother's Old-Fashioned Tea Cakes. For those not familiar with tea cakes, they are almost like a cookie, but they aren't. They are almost like a scone, but they aren't. And they are almost like a shortbread, but they aren't. They are a textural mixture of all three. Lightly sweet and crumbly, these are great with hot tea or coffee. I converted her recipe to be keto friendly and added the zesty flavors of lemon and lime.

FOR THE TEA CAKES

½ cup unsalted butter, at room temperature
⅓ cup powdered erythritol
2 eggs
3 tablespoons lemon juice
½ teaspoon vanilla extract
2¼ cup almond flour, sifted

½ cup oat fiber
1½ teaspoons baking powder

FOR THE GLAZE

⅓ cup plus 1 tablespoon powdered erythritol
2 tablespoons lime juice
Grated zest of 1 lime

TO MAKE THE TEA CAKES

1. Preheat the oven to 350°F. Line a baking sheet with parchment paper.

2. In a large bowl, cream the butter and erythritol for 3 to 4 minutes with a hand mixer until light and fluffy.

3. Add the eggs one at a time and mix thoroughly after each addition.

4. Add the lemon juice and vanilla. Mix well.

5. In a separate bowl, whisk together the almond flour, oat fiber, and baking powder until combined.

6. Slowly add the dry ingredients to the wet ingredients and mix on medium speed for a minute.

7. Using a 1-ounce or 2-tablespoon portion scoop, place scoops of batter on the prepared baking sheet about 3 inches apart. Cover with more parchment paper and use a second baking sheet to press down on the cakes until they are ½-inch thick. Place the baking sheet of tea cakes in the refrigerator for 15 minutes.

8. Bake for 15 minutes. The tea cakes should not be browned on top. Remove from the oven, and using a spatula, carefully move each cake to a cooling rack.

TO MAKE THE GLAZE

9. In a small bowl, whisk together the erythritol and lime juice until a moderately thick glaze forms.

10. Transfer the glaze to a small zip-top bag. Press the glaze into a bottom corner of the bag, cut off a small portion of the corner plastic, and gently squeeze the glaze out across all the cookies.

11. Sprinkle with the lime zest and allow the cookies and glaze to completely cool before storing.

Per serving: Calories: 96; Total Fat: 9g; Total Carbs: 4g; Fiber: 1g; Net Carbs: 3g; Protein: 3g; Erythritol: 7g
Macronutrients: Fat: 79%; Protein: 9%; Carbs: 12%

Summer Squash Mock Apple Crumble

Serves 8
Prep time: 10 minutes

Cook time: 1 hour 5 minutes
Total time: 1 hour 15 minutes

The fall flavors of apple pie are captured beautifully in this mock apple crumble. This recipe uses yellow summer squash as a replacement for apples, and I can tell you that it is very convincing. The warm flavors of cinnamon, nutmeg, and ginger round out the flavors of the filling. The nutty crumb topping is particularly nice if you use the golden or "brown sugar" version of erythritol, which adds the depth of flavor found in brown sugar. Serve with a dollop of whipped cream or a small scoop of keto vanilla ice cream.

FOR THE FILLING

8 tablespoons (1 stick) butter
⅓ cup powdered erythritol
4 tablespoons lemon juice
1½ teaspoons ground cinnamon
1 teaspoon ground nutmeg
½ teaspoon ground ginger
6 cups yellow summer squash, cut into ½-inch pieces
2 teaspoons vanilla extract
Grated zest of 1 lemon (1 heaping tablespoon)

FOR THE CRUMBLE

1¼ cups almond flour
⅓ cup walnuts, chopped
⅓ cup golden erythritol
1 teaspoon ground cinnamon
½ teaspoon ground nutmeg
5 tablespoons plus 1 teaspoon butter, melted

TO MAKE THE FILLING

1. In a large saucepan or pot over medium heat, melt the butter and add the erythritol, lemon juice, cinnamon, nutmeg, and ginger. Whisk to combine well and melt the sweetener.

2. Add the squash. Simmer on medium-low heat for 35 minutes, stirring occasionally.

3. Remove the pot from the heat and stir in the vanilla and lemon zest. Set aside.

4. Preheat the oven to 350°F. Butter a 9-by-9-inch baking dish.

TO MAKE THE CRUMBLE

5. In a large bowl, combine the almond flour, walnuts, erythritol, cinnamon, and nutmeg. Pour over the melted butter and stir well.

6. Pour the squash mixture into the buttered baking dish. Evenly spread the crumb topping over the squash. Gently press down to lightly pack the crumb topping.

7. Bake for 30 minutes or until the top is lightly golden brown.

8. Allow to cool before serving.

> SUBSTITUTION TIP: This dessert also works well with chopped zucchini instead of squash, or even a combination of the two. Both are easily interchangeable.

Per serving: Calories: 286; Total Fat: 28g; Total Carbs: 7g; Fiber: 3g; Net Carbs: 4g; Protein: 4g; Erythritol: 16g
Macronutrients: Fat: 86%; Protein: 5%; Carbs: 9%

Cinnamon Coffee Cake

Serves 16
Prep time: 10 minutes

Cook time: 40 minutes
Total time: 50 minutes

This keto version of coffee cake holds true to the original with a moist, lightly flavored cinnamon cake covered in a hearty, nut-filled crumble. The crumble is my favorite part of coffee cake, so I've put a layer in the middle of the cake as well as on top. This recipe is heavy on ingredients, but the number of portions makes it worthwhile to make ahead for a large gathering, or for freezing and storing for when the sweet-tooth cravings hit.

FOR THE CAKE

2 cups almond flour
½ cup powdered erythritol
2 teaspoons baking powder
1 teaspoon ground cinnamon
¼ teaspoon ground nutmeg
Pinch salt
3 eggs
5 tablespoons butter, at room
   temperature
½ cup full-fat sour cream

¼ cup unsweetened almond milk
1 teaspoon vanilla extract

FOR THE CINNAMON CRUMBLE

2 cups almond flour
¼ cup powdered erythritol
2 teaspoons ground cinnamon
¼ teaspoon ground nutmeg
¼ teaspoon salt
½ cup chopped walnuts
½ cup butter, melted

TO MAKE THE CAKE

1. Preheat the oven to 350°F. Butter a 9-by-9-inch baking dish or line it with parchment paper.

2. Sift the almond flour, erythritol, baking powder, cinnamon, nutmeg, and salt into a large bowl and whisk to combine.

3. In a mixing bowl, use a hand mixer or whisk to cream together the eggs and butter until fluffy. Add the sour cream, almond milk, and vanilla. Mix to combine.

4. Slowly add the dry ingredients and mix to combine.

TO MAKE THE CINNAMON CRUMBLE

5. In a large bowl, combine the almond flour, erythritol, cinnamon, nutmeg, salt, and walnuts, and whisk to combine. Add the butter and mix.

6. Pour half of the cake batter into the prepared baking dish. Sprinkle half of the crumble on top of the batter. Add the rest of the cake batter, then sprinkle the remaining crumble on top. Very gently press the crumble into the batter.

7. Bake for 35 to 40 minutes or until a toothpick inserted comes out clean. Halfway through cooking, loosely cover the dish with aluminum foil to prevent the crumble from burning.

8. Allow to cool and serve.

SUBSTITUTION TIP: Swap out the chopped walnuts for your favorite nuts. I like to use a mixture of walnuts and pecans, but the recipe also works with chopped almonds or macadamia nuts. Check the prices of nuts when you purchase and buy what's on sale.

Per serving: Calories: 234; Total Fat: 22g; Total Carbs: 5g; Fiber: 3g; Net Carbs: 2g; Protein: 5g; Erythritol: 9g
Macronutrients: Fat: 82%; Protein: 9%; Carbs: 9%

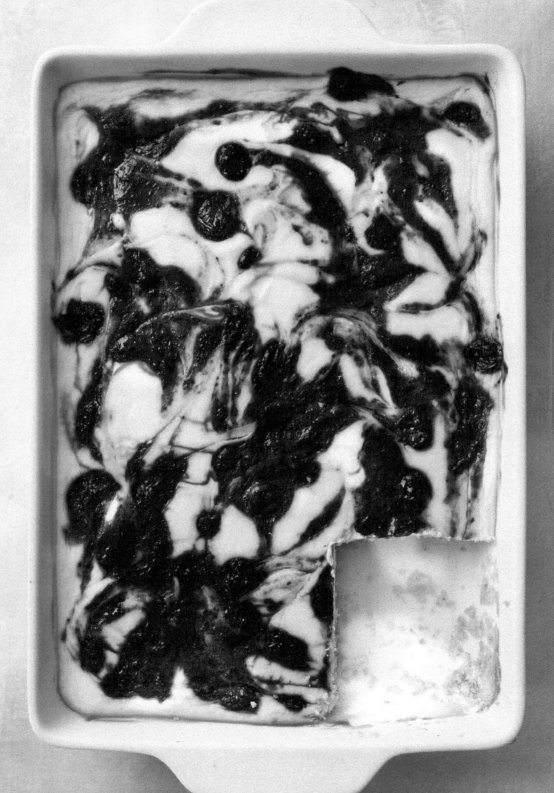

Blueberry Cheesecake Bars

Serves 12
Prep time: 15 minutes

Cook time: 40 minutes
Total time: 55 minutes

This recipe brings the flavor and creamy texture of cheesecake to an easy-to-eat and easy-to-make dessert. The berry swirl looks beautiful and adds the delicious, sweet flavor and healthy anthocyanins berries supply. If you're wanting a little crunch, add ½ cup of finely chopped pecans to the crust mixture. These bars store well in the refrigerator, but it's best to eat them within a week. Freezing can cause the cream cheese to break.

FOR THE BLUEBERRY COMPOTE

2 cups blueberries, fresh or frozen
2 teaspoons powdered erythritol
2 tablespoons lemon juice
Grated zest of 1 lemon (1 heaping
  tablespoon)

FOR THE CRUST

2 cups almond flour

2 teaspoons powdered erythritol
½ teaspoon ground cinnamon
12 tablespoons (1½ sticks) butter, melted

FOR THE FILLING

16 ounces cream cheese, at room
  temperature
2 eggs, at room temperature
½ cup powdered erythritol
2 teaspoons vanilla extract

TO MAKE THE BLUEBERRY COMPOTE

In a small saucepan, combine all the ingredients and cook over medium heat for 15 minutes, stirring occasionally.

TO MAKE THE CRUST

1. While the compote cooks, preheat the oven to 350°F, and butter a 9-by-13-inch baking dish.

2. In a large bowl, combine all the ingredients and mix well. Press the mixture into the buttered baking dish to make a crust. Bake at 350°F for 12 minutes. Remove from the oven.

TO MAKE THE FILLING

3. In a large mixing bowl, combine all the ingredients and use a hand mixer to mix well. The cheesecake filling should be light and fluffy, but don't overmix.

4. Pour the filling into the prebaked crust and use a spatula to spread it evenly. ▶

Blueberry Cheesecake Bars CONTINUED

5. Spoon the blueberry compote over the top of the filling. Use a knife to swirl the compote into the filling.

6. Bake for 35 to 40 minutes or until the cheesecake is set. When cool, chill in the refrigerator for at least 1 hour to set up. Cut and serve.

SUBSTITUTION TIP: Try this recipe with your favorite berries. Blackberries, strawberries, blueberries, or a frozen berry medley work great.

Per serving: Calories: 324; Total Fat: 31g; Total Carbs: 8g; Fiber: 2g; Net Carbs: 6g; Protein: 6g; Erythritol: 9g
Macronutrients: Fat: 83%; Protein: 7%; Carbs: 10%

Classic Chocolate Chip Cookies

Makes 18
Prep time: 15 minutes

Cook time: 10 minutes
Total time: 25 minutes

Sugar-free chocolate chips are available in many grocery stores. I particularly like the brands Lily's Chocolate and Bake Believe. If you can't find them in the baking aisle, head over to the candy aisle with the gourmet chocolate bars and look for Lily's chocolate bars. These can be chopped into chip-size pieces.

1¼ cups almond flour
2 tablespoons oat fiber
½ teaspoon baking powder
½ teaspoon salt
½ cup butter, at room temperature

½ cup golden erythritol sweetener
1 egg
2 teaspoons vanilla extract
⅓ cup sugar-free chocolate chips

1. Preheat the oven to 350°F. Line a large baking sheet with parchment paper.

2. In a medium bowl, sift together the flour, oat fiber, baking powder, and salt. Whisk to combine.

3. In a large mixing bowl, use a hand mixer to cream together the butter and erythritol until the sweetener has dissolved and the butter is fluffy.

4. Add the egg and vanilla and continue to beat for 3 to 4 minutes at high speed until light and fluffy.

5. Incorporate the dry ingredients and mix until just combined.

6. Using a rubber spatula, fold in the chocolate chips.

7. Use a spoon to make 9 cookies (about half the dough) on the baking sheet. Gently press the dough to lightly flatten them. (They will spread when cooked, so don't flatten them too much.)

8. Bake for 10 minutes, turning the baking sheet halfway through.

9. Cook the second batch when the baking sheet has fully cooled. Allow to cool and then serve.

METHOD TIP: If you have a stand mixer, use the dough paddle on medium-high speed to easily and quickly work the butter and sugar into a fluffy batter.

Per serving: Calories: 80; Total Fat: 8g; Total Carbs: 2g; Fiber: 1g; Net Carbs: 1g; Protein: 2g; Erythritol: 5g
Macronutrients: Fat: 86%; Protein: 7%; Carbs: 7%

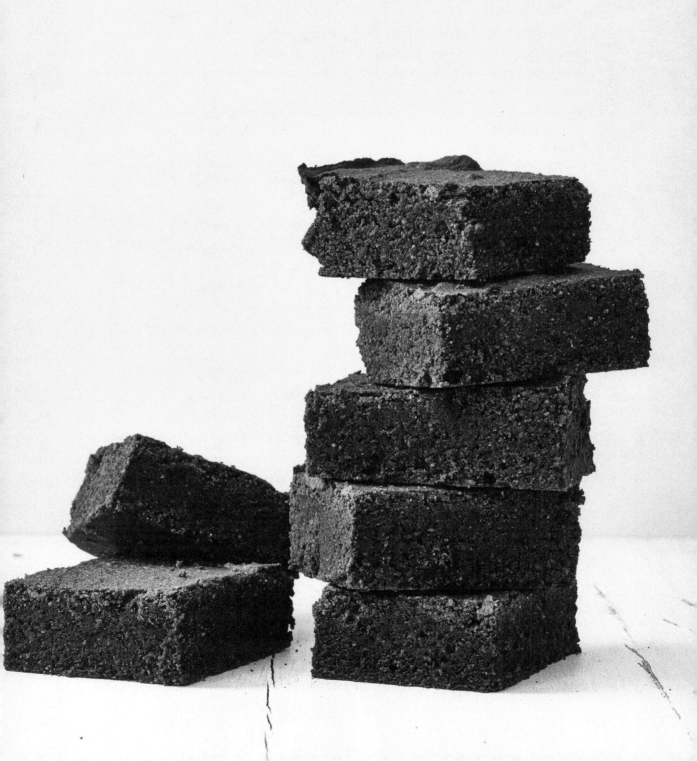

Classic Chocolate Brownies

Serves 12
Prep time: 10 minutes

Cook time: 30 minutes
Total time: 40 minutes

As a kid, one of the first things I learned to bake for myself was brownies from a box. My older brother would break out the baking pan after dinner had been put away and make brownies for family movie night. It wasn't too many years later that he moved off to college and I started making those Duncan Hines or Betty Crocker brownies myself. This keto version is similar in texture and flavor to the boxed brownie mix that I grew up loving—and they really hit the spot if you're fighting the sweet tooth monster.

8 tablespoons (1 stick) butter, plus more for greasing
1½ ounces unsweetened Baker's Chocolate
1¼ cups powdered erythritol
7 tablespoons cocoa powder

¼ teaspoon salt
3 eggs, beaten
2 tablespoons water
1½ teaspoons vanilla extract
1¼ cups almond flour

1. Preheat the oven to 350°F. Butter an 8-by-8-inch baking dish.

2. Fill a medium saucepan with 2 inches of water and bring to a simmer over medium heat. Place a large glass bowl over the pot to create a double boiler.

3. Put the butter and chocolate in the bowl and stir until melted. Add the erythritol, cocoa powder, and salt, and whisk until the sweetener is dissolved. Remove from the heat.

4. Allow to cool for a few minutes. Whisk in the eggs a little at a time. Whisk in the water and vanilla.

5. Gradually add the almond flour and stir to combine.

6. Pour the batter into the baking dish and use a rubber spatula to spread it out evenly.

7. Bake for about 30 minutes or until a toothpick inserted comes out clean. Allow to cool completely before cutting and serving.

METHOD TIP: You can melt the butter and chocolate in a microwave. Soften them on medium power for 1 minute and stir. Repeat until both are melted, then continue with the recipe as written.

Per serving: Calories: 158; Total Fat: 15g; Total Carbs: 4g; Fiber: 2g; Net Carbs: 2g; Protein: 4g; Erythritol: 20g
Macronutrients: Fat: 82%; Protein: 10%; Carbs: 8%

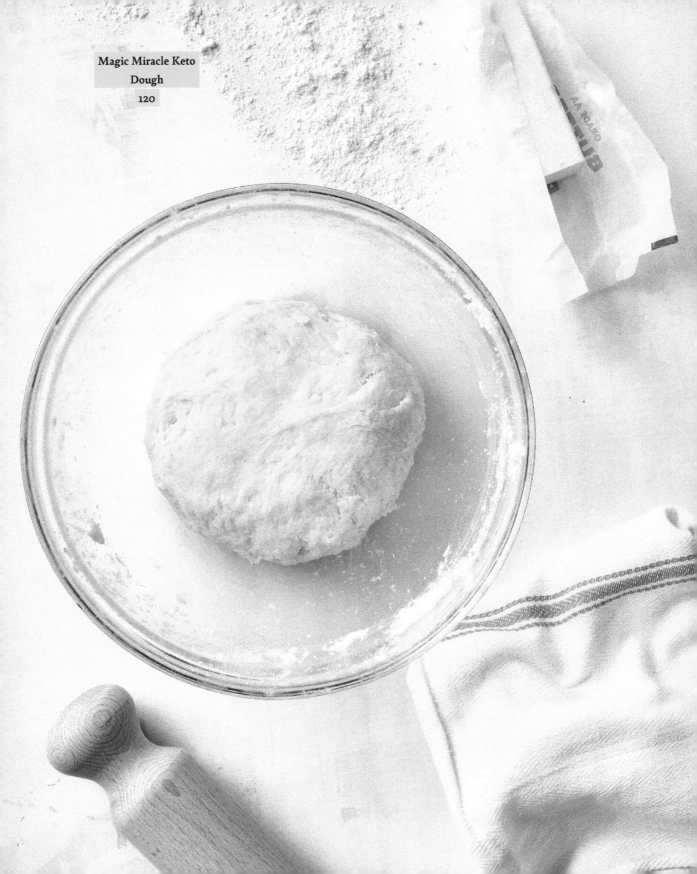

CHAPTER 8

Keto Staples

Magic Miracle Keto Dough 120

Beef Bone Broth 122

Chicken Bone Broth 124

Vegetable Broth 125

Cheese Crisps 127

Easy Guacamole 128

Almond Flour Crackers 129

Chocolate Almond Fat
Bombs 131

Keto Butter Coffee 132

Magic Miracle Keto Dough

Serves 6 to 8　　　　　　　　　　　**Cook time:** 15 minutes
Prep time: 10 minutes　　　　　　　**Total time:** 25 minutes

This recipe is a variation of what is lovingly referred to by the keto community as "fathead dough" (based upon the documentary *Fathead*). It has since been modified by countless cooks and recipe developers to create all manner of baked goods. This version uses coconut flour. I feel it gives the best flavor and texture, plus coconut flour is lower in carbs and calories than almond flour, uses less flour overall, and costs less. It can be used for pizza crust, bread sticks, bagels, cinnamon rolls, and many other quick breads. I've included a few variations so you can see how versatile this recipe is.

½ cup coconut flour
2 teaspoons baking powder
2½ cups shredded mozzarella cheese

2 ounces full-fat cream cheese
3 large eggs, beaten
2 tablespoons butter, melted

1. Preheat the oven to 350°F and line a baking sheet with parchment paper.

2. Sift together the coconut flour and baking powder in a small bowl.

3. In a separate bowl, melt the mozzarella and cream cheese in the microwave on high power for 1 minute. Stir. Zap it on high for another minute. Stir.

4. Using damp hands or a dough hook, mix in the eggs, butter, and flour mixture until a dough is formed. The dough should be a bit wet and sticky.

FOR PIZZA CRUST

1. Place a piece of parchment paper on the countertop and turn out the dough. Place another piece of parchment paper on top and roll the dough into a thin rectangle. Transfer the bottom parchment paper and dough to a baking sheet.

2. Bake at 350°F for 10 to 15 minutes, until slightly browned. Cover with sauce, toppings, and cheese and bake until melted and bubbly.

FOR BAGELS

1. Divide the dough into 8 equal portions. Roll the portions between your hands into 8-inch logs. With each log, make a loose bagel shape and pinch the ends together. Place on a parchment paper–lined baking sheet.

2. Bake at 350°F for 15 minutes or until the bagels are fluffy and browned. Slice and serve.

FOR CHEESY GARLIC BREAD STICKS

1. Place a piece of parchment paper on the countertop and turn out the dough. Place another piece of parchment paper on top and roll the dough into a rectangle about 1 inch thick. Transfer the bottom parchment paper and dough to a baking sheet.

2. Bake at 350°F for 10 to 15 minutes, until slightly browned. Brush with melted garlic butter, sprinkle lightly with your favorite cheese, and bake until melted.

FOR CINNAMON ROLLS

1. Place a piece of parchment paper on the countertop and turn out the dough. Place another piece of parchment paper on top and roll the dough into a rectangle about 1 inch thick.

2. In a small bowl, combine ⅓ cup of golden erythritol, ¼ cup of chopped pecans, and 1½ teaspoons of ground cinnamon. Mix well. Spread 3 tablespoons of room-temperature butter on the dough and evenly sprinkle with the cinnamon-sugar mixture. Lightly pat it with your fingertips.

3. Starting at the long end, gently roll the dough into a log. Slice into 12 even rolls and place them cut-side up in a 9-by-13-inch baking dish. Bake for 18 to 20 minutes, until lightly browned.

4. Make a quick icing by whisking together 2 tablespoons of room-temperature cream cheese, 2 tablespoons of melted butter, and ¼ cup of powdered erythritol. Spread over the warm rolls and serve.

> **METHOD TIP:** You can melt the mozzarella and cream cheese in a double boiler. Set a bowl over a saucepan on medium-high heat filled with 2 inches of water. Allow the cheeses to gently melt, then remove from the heat.

Per serving: Calories: 281; Total Fat: 21g; Total Carbs: 7g; Fiber: 3g; Net Carbs: 4g; Protein: 16g
Macronutrients: Fat: 67%; Protein: 23%; Carbs: 10%

Beef Bone Broth

Serves 6 to 8　　　　　　　　　　**Cook time:** 12 to 24 hours
Prep time: 10 minutes　　　　　　**Total time:** 12 to 24 hours

Bone broth is a staple of many keto dieters. We use it in recipes and also sip this intense, deeply flavored broth in a mug for the essential collagen, vitamins, minerals, and electrolytes. In addition to a very lengthy cook time at low heat, this recipe calls for apple cider vinegar, which breaks down the collagen within the bones to aid in the extraction. When searching for bones, price will depend on what's in stock and freshest. I often shop in the frozen section where beef bones are sold specifically for soup making. These are a great savings over fresh bones. Ask the butcher where the frozen beef bones are located.

---

3 to 4 pounds beef bones (oxtails, neck bones, short ribs)
1 tablespoon olive oil
2 medium carrots, peeled and coarsely chopped
2 celery stalks, coarsely chopped

1 medium white onion, unpeeled, quartered
4 garlic cloves, peeled and smashed
3 bay leaves
2 tablespoons apple cider vinegar
1 tablespoon sea salt
10 cups water

1. Preheat the oven to 400°F. Line a baking sheet with aluminum foil.

2. Place the beef bones on the baking sheet and drizzle with the olive oil.

3. Roast for 1 hour. Turn the bones over halfway through.

4. Continue with one of the following cooking options: stovetop, slow cooker, or multicooker.

5. Once cooked, remove the bones from the pot or cooker with tongs. Strain the broth into a large bowl to remove the vegetables. Allow to cool to room temperature, then refrigerate. Once chilled, scrape off the separated fat, if desired.

STOVETOP OPTION

1. In a large stockpot with a lid, combine the roasted bones and the carrots, celery, onion, garlic, bay leaves, vinegar, and sea salt. Completely cover with the water.

2. Turn the heat to high and bring to a boil. Reduce the heat to low, cover, and simmer for 8 to 12 hours.

SLOW COOKER OPTION

1. In a large slow cooker, combine the roasted bones and the carrots, celery, onion, garlic, bay leaves, vinegar, and sea salt. Completely cover with the water.

2. Turn to the high setting. When it starts to boil, turn to the low setting, secure the lid, and cook for 18 to 24 hours.

MULTICOOKER OPTION

1. Combine the roasted beef bones and the carrots, celery, onion, garlic, bay leaves, vinegar, and sea salt in the multicooker. Completely cover with the water.

2. Seal the lid and turn the manual setting to high. Set the timer for 120 minutes. Allow a natural release of pressure.

> **BATCH-COOKING TIP:** After refrigerating, spoon off any excess fat that has risen to the top, portion in zip-top freezer bags or freezer-safe containers, and store in the freezer for up to 5 months.

Per serving: Calories: 40; Total Fat: 0g; Total Carbs: 0g; Fiber: 0g; Net Carbs: 0g; Protein: 10g
Macronutrients: Fat: 5%; Protein: 95%; Carbs: 0%

Chicken Bone Broth

SUPER SAVER

Serves 6 to 8
Prep time: 10 minutes

Cook time: 12 to 24 hours
Total time: 12 to 24 hours

All the statements and qualifications that apply to the Beef Bone Broth recipe (page 122) apply to chicken bone broth. This broth can be made from the carcass of a couple of roasted chickens, or you can use some chicken wings or even chicken feet.

2 chicken carcasses, meat removed, or 2 pounds chicken wings or feet
2 medium carrots, peeled and coarsely chopped
2 celery stalks, coarsely chopped
1 medium white onion, unpeeled, quartered
4 garlic cloves, peeled and smashed

3 bay leaves
3 or 4 fresh herb sprigs (e.g., tarragon or rosemary)
2 tablespoons apple cider vinegar
1 tablespoon sea salt
10 cups water

STOVETOP OPTION

1. In a large stockpot with a lid, combine the bones, carrots, celery, onion, garlic, bay leaves, herbs, vinegar, and salt. Completely cover with the water.

2. Turn the heat to high and bring to a boil. Reduce the heat to low, cover, and simmer for 8 to 12 hours.

SLOW COOKER OPTION

1. In a large slow cooker, combine the bones, carrots, celery, onion, garlic, bay leaves, herbs, vinegar, and salt. Completely cover with the water.

2. Turn to the high setting. When it starts to boil, turn to the low setting, secure the lid, and cook for 18 to 24 hours.

MULTICOOKER OPTION

1. Combine the bones, carrots, celery, onion, garlic, bay leaves, herbs, vinegar, and salt in the multicooker. Completely cover with the water.

2. Seal the lid and turn the manual setting to high. Set the timer for 120 minutes. Allow a natural release of pressure.

INGREDIENT TIP: If you don't have a rotisserie chicken carcass, head to the cold section of the grocery deli, where you can pick up one left over from the day before at half the price.

Per serving: Calories: 45; Total Fat: 0g; Total Carbs: 1g; Fiber: 0g; Net Carbs: 1g; Protein: 10g
Macronutrients: Fat: 4%; Protein: 91%; Carbs: 5%

Vegetable Broth

Serves 6 to 8

Prep time: 5 minutes

Cook time: 1 hour

Total time: 1 hour 5 minutes

Vegetable broth doesn't contain the natural fats and collagen that beef or chicken bone broths do. But many people enjoy cooking with or just sipping vegetable broth. There are even vegan keto followers who use vegetable stock in place of animal-based broths. This recipe uses aromatics that can contain a good bit of natural sugars, but most of that is discarded at the end of cooking. Some natural sugars dissolve into the broth, but they are minimal.

3 leeks

2 tablespoons olive oil

3 carrots, peeled and coarsely chopped

3 celery stalks

1 medium yellow onion, unpeeled, quartered

½ cup sliced mushrooms

4 garlic cloves, peeled and smashed

2 teaspoons dried thyme

2 bay leaves

3 teaspoons salt

10 whole peppercorns

Leftover vegetable scraps (optional)

10 cups water

1. Halve the leeks lengthwise and rinse under running water to remove any sand. Coarsely chop them.

2. In a large stockpot over medium-high heat, heat the olive oil.

3. When the oil is hot, add the leeks, carrots, celery, onion, mushrooms, garlic, and thyme. Sauté for 8 to 10 minutes until there is light browning on the vegetables.

4. Add the bay leaves, salt, peppercorns, and vegetable scraps (if using), and cover with the water.

5. Turn the heat to high and bring to a boil. Reduce the heat to low, cover the pot, and cook for 1 hour.

6. Strain into a bowl. Allow to cool. Refrigerate for up to 5 days or portion and freeze.

INGREDIENT TIP: Vegetable broth (and really any broth) is a great way to use vegetable scraps. If you plan to make veggie broth, save any vegetable cuttings, stems, or herbs in a zip-top bag in the refrigerator. Add these to the other vegetables to really round out the flavor.

Per serving: Calories: 15; Total Fat: 0g; Total Carbs: 3g; Fiber: 1g; Net Carbs: 2g; Protein: 1g
Macronutrients: Fat: 0%; Protein: 24%; Carbs: 76%

Cheese Crisps

Serves 6
Prep time: 5 minutes

Cook time: 10 minutes
Total time: 15 minutes

These crispy little crackers are a true keto staple. They are great as a snack by themselves, served with your favorite dip, or even as croutons in a big salad. The crackers can be made with most hard cheeses (Gouda, Swiss, Parmesan, etc.) but they won't work with soft "melting" cheeses, such as mozzarella, or processed cheese, such as American slices.

6 slices thin deli-style cheddar cheese
Pinch paprika

Pinch Italian seasoning

1. Preheat the oven to 375°F. Line two baking sheets with parchment paper. (Or make in batches, as these crackers spread significantly while baking.)

2. Cut the cheese slices into quarters and place on the baking sheets.

3. Lightly sprinkle with paprika and Italian seasoning.

4. Bake for 7 to 8 minutes or until bubbly.

5. Remove from the oven and allow to cool for 10 minutes to get crispy. Blot with a paper towel to remove excess oil. Serve immediately or allow to cool and store in a zip-top bag with a folded paper towel to remove any excess oil and moisture.

INGREDIENT TIP: This recipe also works with shredded cheese. Just make small mounds of shredded cheese on the parchment paper and cook as directed.

Per serving: Calories: 77; Total Fat: 6g; Total Carbs: 0g; Fiber: 0g; Net Carbs: 0g; Protein: 5g
Macronutrients: Fat: 75%; Protein: 24%; Carbs: 1%

Easy Guacamole

Serves 6
Prep time: 10 minutes

Total time: 10 minutes

Fresh, homemade guacamole made from perfectly ripe avocados is a real treat. The healthy fat and high fiber content make this a wonderful keto condiment for many dishes, or a dip for Almond Flour Crackers (page 129).

4 avocados
Juice of 1 lime
¼ cup minced red onion
1 garlic clove, minced

3 cherry tomatoes, finely chopped
½ teaspoon salt
¼ teaspoon freshly ground black pepper
¼ teaspoon chili powder

1. Halve the avocados and remove the pits. Use a spoon to scoop the avocado flesh into a medium bowl.

2. Pour the lime juice over the avocado flesh.

3. Use a fork to mash the avocado to your desired consistency.

4. Add the onion, garlic, tomatoes, salt, pepper, and chili powder, and stir to combine.

5. Serve immediately. Cover leftovers tightly with cling wrap and refrigerate for up to 3 days.

Per serving: Calories: 250; Total Fat: 20g; Total Carbs: 18g; Fiber: 12g; Net Carbs: 6g; Protein: 5g
Macronutrients: Fat: 68%; Protein: 7%; Carbs: 25%

Almond Flour Crackers

Serves 6
Prep time: 5 minutes

Cook time: 25 minutes
Total time: 30 minutes

In the keto world, baking crispy crackers without using lots of seeds can be difficult to pull off. But fear not, this recipe makes perfect little crunchy crackers that are great for snacking or dipping. Like a few other recipes in this book, I recommend using powdered Parmesan cheese in a can. This product is finely ground like a flour, so it behaves like a flour when cooked.

1 cup blanched almond flour
¼ cup powdered Parmesan cheese in a can
4 tablespoons water

½ teaspoon garlic powder
½ teaspoon Italian seasoning
Coarse sea salt

1. Preheat the oven to 350°F.

2. In a medium bowl, combine the flour, Parmesan, water, garlic powder, and Italian seasoning, and stir to form a dough.

3. Place the dough between two pieces of parchment paper. Use a rolling pin or wine bottle to roll the dough into a thin rectangle slightly smaller than the baking sheet.

4. Remove the top piece of parchment paper. Lift the bottom parchment paper and transfer it to the baking sheet.

5. Lightly sprinkle coarse salt over the dough, and gently press it in.

6. Using a pizza wheel or sharp knife, cut the dough into 1-inch squares. Use a toothpick to create a small hole in the center of each cracker.

7. Bake for about 25 minutes or until lightly browned. Allow to cool on a wire rack, then break the crackers apart. Store for up to 1 week in the pantry in a zip-top bag.

INGREDIENT TIP: For best results, this recipe must be made with finely ground almond flour from blanched almonds, *not* coarse almond meal.

Per serving: Calories: 87; Total Fat: 7g; Total Carbs: 3g; Fiber: 2g; Net Carbs: 1g; Protein: 4g
Macronutrients: Fat: 70%; Protein: 16%; Carbs: 14%

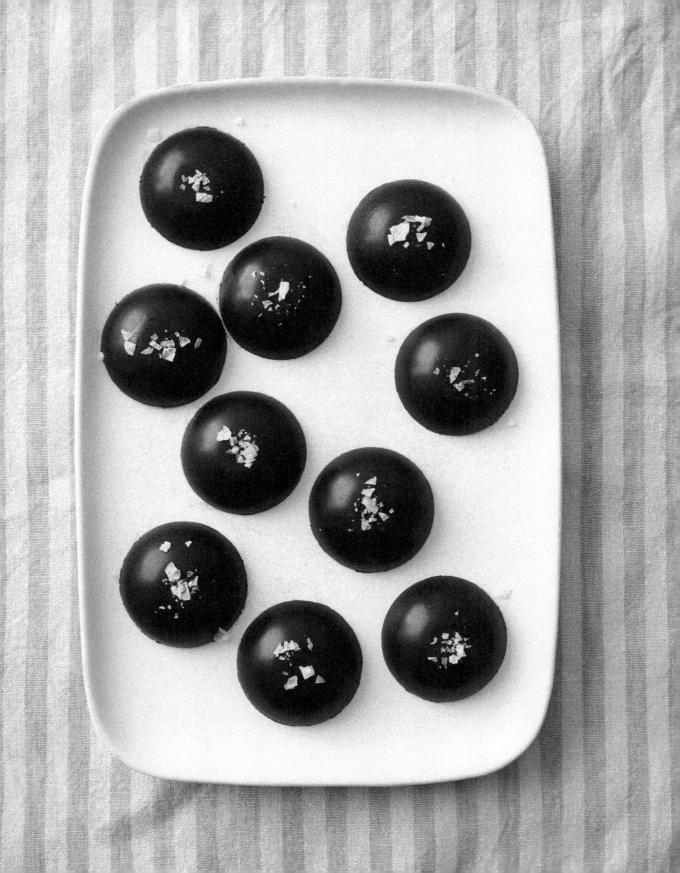

Chocolate Almond Fat Bombs

Makes 12　　　　　　　　　　　　**Cook time:** 5 minutes
Prep time: 5 minutes　　　　　　**Total time:** 10 minutes

Fat bombs are exactly what the name implies: a large serving of fat to help you meet your fat macros for the day. They can be sweet or savory, but this recipe is for sweet, chocolatey, nut-filled fat bombs. These work best in a silicone candy mold for 2-inch candies but can also be made in paper mini muffin liners on a baking sheet. The coconut oil melts at anything slightly over room temperature, so store these bombs in the refrigerator or freeze them.

12 tablespoons coconut oil
6 tablespoons cocoa powder
2 tablespoons powdered erythritol

½ teaspoon vanilla extract
24 whole raw almonds
Coarse sea salt

1. Place 12 candy molds or miniature muffin tin liners on a large baking sheet.
2. In a small saucepan over medium heat, melt the coconut oil.
3. Add the cocoa powder, erythritol, and vanilla, and whisk well to combine.
4. Spoon the mixture into the candy molds. Drop 2 almonds into each mold. Refrigerate until the chocolate is set.
5. Remove the bombs from the molds and press a pinch of coarse sea salt onto the top of each chocolate.
6. Store in a zip-top bag in the refrigerator for up to 1 week, or in the freezer for up to 3 months.

SUBSTITUTION TIP: Use any low-carb nut you like in place of the almonds. Try walnuts, pecans, hazelnuts, or macadamia nuts.

Per serving: Calories: 138; Total Fat: 15g; Total Carbs: 2g; Fiber: 1g; Net Carbs: 1g; Protein: 1g; Erythritol: 4g
Macronutrients: Fat: 95%; Protein: 2%; Carbs: 3%

Keto Butter Coffee

Serves 2
Prep time: 5 minutes

Total time: 5 minutes

Keto butter coffee is a great way to start the day. The healthy fats from the butter, cream, and coconut oil help meet your fat macros, and the MCT (medium chain triglycerides) in the coconut oil, along with the caffeine from the coffee, help keep you alert and energized. But this creamy, frothy beverage can't be stirred in a mug, because that just leads to coffee with a big oil slick; it must be either mixed with a blender or in a shaker cup used for making protein shakes. Butter coffee is best made fresh and doesn't reheat well, so if you're cooking for a crowd, make it in small batches (this recipe is for two servings) to ensure the butter is fully incorporated into the coffee without overcrowding a dangerously hot blender.

---

16 ounces freshly brewed hot coffee
¼ cup heavy cream
1 tablespoon unsalted butter
1 tablespoon coconut oil

5 drops stevia or sweetener of choice
1 teaspoon cocoa powder or ½ teaspoon
　ground cinnamon (optional)

Combine all the ingredients in a blender, and blend until creamy and frothy, about 20 seconds. Pour into 2 coffee cups and serve.

Per serving: Calories: 212; Total Fat: 24g; Total Carbs: 1g; Fiber: 0g; Net Carbs: 1g; Protein: 1g; Erythritol: 2g
Macronutrients: Fat: 97%; Protein: 1%; Carbs: 2

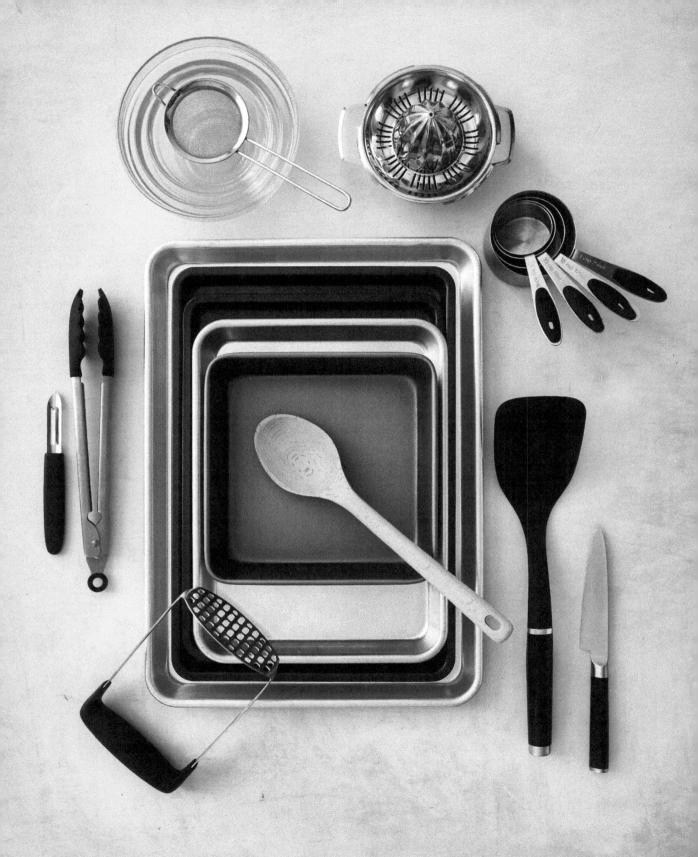

Measurement Conversions

VOLUME EQUIVALENTS (LIQUID)

US STANDARD	US STANDARD (OUNCES)	METRIC (APPROXIMATE)
2 tablespoons	1 fl. oz.	30 mL
¼ cup	2 fl. oz.	60 mL
½ cup	4 fl. oz.	120 mL
1 cup	8 fl. oz.	240 mL
1½ cups	12 fl. oz.	355 mL
2 cups or 1 pint	16 fl. oz.	475 mL
4 cups or 1 quart	32 fl. oz.	1 L
1 gallon	128 fl. oz.	4 L

OVEN TEMPERATURES

FAHRENHEIT (F)	CELSIUS (C) (APPROXIMATE)
250°F	120°C
300°F	150°C
325°F	165°C
350°F	180°C
375°F	190°C
400°F	200°C
425°F	220°C
450°F	230°C

VOLUME EQUIVALENTS (DRY)

US STANDARD	METRIC (APPROXIMATE)
⅛ teaspoon	0.5 mL
¼ teaspoon	1 mL
½ teaspoon	2 mL
¾ teaspoon	4 mL
1 teaspoon	5 mL
1 tablespoon	15 mL
¼ cup	59 mL
⅓ cup	79 mL
½ cup	118 mL
⅔ cup	156 mL
¾ cup	177 mL
1 cup	235 mL
2 cups or 1 pint	475 mL
3 cups	700 mL
4 cups or 1 quart	1 L

WEIGHT EQUIVALENTS

US STANDARD	METRIC (APPROXIMATE)
½ ounce	15 g
1 ounce	30 g
2 ounces	60 g
4 ounces	115 g
8 ounces	225 g
12 ounces	340 g
16 ounces or 1 pound	455 g

Index

A

Almond Flour Crackers, 129
Almonds
    Chocolate Almond
        Fat Bombs, 131
    Roasted Green Bean
        Almandine with Blistered
        Tomatoes, 48
Asparagus, Bacon-Wrapped, 47
Avocados
    Baked Egg Avocado
        Boats, 24
    Easy Guacamole, 128

B

Bacon
    Bacon Broccoli Crustless
        Quiche Cups, 15
    Bacon-Wrapped
        Asparagus, 47
    Classic Cobb Salad, 41
    Spinach Salad with Warm
        Bacon Dressing, 39
Bagels, 120
Batch-and-freeze cooking, 7–8
Beef
    Beef Bone Broth, 122–123
    Beef Empanadas, 87
    Cheesesteak-Stuffed
        Bell Peppers, 85
    Easy Mississippi Pot
        Roast, 82
    Keto Beef Chili, 35
    Mom's Pot Roast with
        Gravy and Radish
        "Potatoes," 98–99
    Pan-Seared Hanger
        Steak with Easy Herb
        Cream Sauce, 83
    Salisbury Steak with
        Mushroom Gravy, 88–89

Shepherd's Pie, 90–91
    Southwest-Style Fajita
        Bowls, 100–101
Bell peppers
    Cheesesteak-Stuffed
        Bell Peppers, 85
    Southwest-Style Fajita
        Bowls, 100–101
Blueberries
    Blueberry Cheesecake
        Bars, 113–114
    Keto Blueberry Pancakes, 20
Bowls
    Breakfast Burrito Bowl, 17
    Egg Roll in a Bowl, 86
    Southwest-Style Fajita
        Bowls, 100–101
Breakfasts
    Bacon Broccoli Crustless
        Quiche Cups, 15
    Baked Egg Avocado
        Boats, 24
    Breakfast Burrito Bowl, 17
    Cheesy Sausage and
        Cabbage Hash, 25
    Classic Diner Hash Browns, 23
    Ham and Cheese Egg Cups, 21
    Keto Blueberry Pancakes, 20
    Overnight Chocolate
        Chia Pudding, 18
    Salmon and Egg Scramble, 19
    Sausage and Cheese
        Frittata, 14
Broccoli
    Bacon Broccoli Crustless
        Quiche Cups, 15
    Broccoli Cheddar Soup, 32
    Crispy Pan-Roasted
        Broccoli, 51
Broths
    Beef Bone Broth, 122–123

Chicken Bone Broth, 124
    Vegetable Broth, 125
Brownies, Classic
    Chocolate, 117
Buffalo Chicken Spaghetti
    Squash, 68–69
Burrito Bowl, Breakfast, 17
Butter Coffee, Keto, 132

C

Cabbage
    Cheesy Sausage and
        Cabbage Hash, 25
    Egg Roll in a Bowl, 86
    Roasted Cabbage Steaks, 55
Cakes
    Cinnamon Coffee
        Cake, 110–111
    Old-Fashioned Lemon-Lime
        Tea Cakes, 106–107
    Quick Pressure Cooker
        Cheesecake, 105
Carbohydrates, 2, 5
Cauliflower
    Coastal Shrimp and
        Cauliflower Grits, 62–63
    Easy Cauliflower Rice, 52
    Loaded Mashed
        Cauliflower, 49
    Shepherd's Pie, 90–91
Cheese
    Broccoli Cheddar Soup, 32
    Cajun Parmesan Pork
        Chops, 93
    Cheese Crisps, 127
    Cheesesteak-Stuffed
        Bell Peppers, 85
    Cheesy Sausage and
        Cabbage Hash, 25
    Garlic Parmesan Chicken
        Wings, 73

Ham and Cheese Egg Cups, 21
Keto Lasagna with Deli
Meat "Noodles," 94–95
Sausage and Cheese
Frittata, 14
Cheesecake
Blueberry Cheesecake
Bars, 113–114
Quick Pressure Cooker
Cheesecake, 105
Chia Pudding, Overnight
Chocolate, 18
Chicken
Baked Lemon Garlic
Chicken, 75
Buffalo Chicken Spaghetti
Squash, 68–69
Chicken and Baby Corn
Chowder, 28–29
Chicken and Sausage
Jambalaya, 77
Chicken Bone Broth, 124
Chicken Divan
Casserole, 66–67
Classic Chicken Salad, 37
Classic Cobb Salad, 41
Coconut Chicken Adobo, 72
Crispy Chicken Tenders, 71
Easy Chicken Alfredo, 76
Garlic Parmesan Chicken
Wings, 73
Keto Lasagna with Deli
Meat "Noodles," 94–95
Southwest-Style
Chicken Soup, 31
Chocolate
Chocolate Almond
Fat Bombs, 131
Classic Chocolate
Brownies, 117
Classic Chocolate Chip
Cookies, 115
Overnight Chocolate
Chia Pudding, 18
Cinnamon Coffee Cake,
110–111

Cinnamon Rolls, 121
Coconut Chicken Adobo, 72
Coffee, Keto Butter, 132
Coffee Cake, Cinnamon,
110–111
Collard Greens, Southern-
Style, 58
Cookies, Classic Chocolate
Chip, 115
Corn Chowder, Chicken
and Baby, 28–29
Crackers
Almond Flour
Crackers, 129
Cheese Crisps, 127
Cream cheese
Blueberry Cheesecake
Bars, 113–114
Quick Pressure Cooker
Cheesecake, 105
Cucumber Tomato
Salad, Cool and
Creamy, 42

D

Desserts
Blueberry Cheesecake
Bars, 113–114
Chocolate Almond
Fat Bombs, 131
Cinnamon Coffee
Cake, 110–111
Classic Chocolate
Brownies, 117
Classic Chocolate Chip
Cookies, 115
Lemon Poppy Seed
Muffins, 104
Old-Fashioned Lemon-Lime
Tea Cakes, 106–107
Quick Pressure Cooker
Cheesecake, 105
Summer Squash Mock Apple
Crumble, 108–109
Dill and Radish "Potato"
Salad, Creamy, 36

Dough, Magic Miracle
Keto, 120–121

E

Egg Roll in a Bowl, 86
Eggs
Bacon Broccoli Crustless
Quiche Cups, 15
Baked Egg Avocado Boats, 24
Classic Cobb Salad, 41
Ham and Cheese Egg
Cups, 21
Salmon and Egg Scramble, 19
Sausage and Cheese
Frittata, 14
Empanadas, Beef, 87
Equipment, 10

F

Fat Bombs, Chocolate
Almond, 131
Fats, 2, 4
Fish and seafood
Classic Tuna Salad, 38
Coastal Shrimp and
Cauliflower Grits, 62–63
Creamy Keto Seafood
Stew, 30
Panfried Tilapia, 70
Salmon and Egg Scramble, 19
Salmon Croquettes, 65

G

Garlic
Baked Lemon Garlic
Chicken, 75
Cheesy Garlic Bread
Sticks, 121
Garlic Parmesan Chicken
Wings, 73
Gravy
Mom's Pot Roast with
Gravy and Radish
"Potatoes," 98–99
Salisbury Steak with
Mushroom Gravy, 88–89

Green Bean Almandine with Blistered Tomatoes, Roasted, 48
Grocery shopping, 6–7
Guacamole, Easy, 128

H

Ham and Cheese Egg Cups, 21
Hash Browns, Classic Diner, 23
Herb Cream Sauce, Pan-Seared Hanger Steak with Easy, 83

I

Ingredient staples, 8–9

K

Kale
  Zuppa Toscana (Sausage and Kale Soup), 33
Ketogenic diet, 2–5
Ketosis, 2–4

L

Lasagna with Deli Meat "Noodles," Keto, 94–95
Lemons
  Baked Lemon Garlic Chicken, 75
  Lemon Poppy Seed Muffins, 104
  Old-Fashioned Lemon-Lime Tea Cakes, 106–107

M

Macronutrients, 2, 4
Meatballs, Sweet and Spicy Turkey, 78–79
Money-saving tips, 5–8
Muffins, Lemon Poppy Seed, 104
Mushroom Gravy, Salisbury Steak with, 88–89

O

Okra, Crispy Pan-Roasted, 59

P

Pancakes, Keto Blueberry, 20
Parmesan cheese
  Cajun Parmesan Pork Chops, 93
  Garlic Parmesan Chicken Wings, 73
Pizza Crust, 120
Poppy Seed Muffins, Lemon, 104
Pork. See also Bacon; Sausage
  Cajun Parmesan Pork Chops, 93
  Classic Pulled Pork, 96–97
  Egg Roll in a Bowl, 86
  Ham and Cheese Egg Cups, 21
Proteins, 2, 5

Q

Quiche Cups, Bacon Broccoli Crustless, 15

R

Radishes
  Classic Diner Hash Browns, 23
  Creamy Dill and Radish "Potato" Salad, 36
  Mom's Pot Roast with Gravy and Radish "Potatoes," 98–99
  Pan-Roasted Red Radish "Potatoes," 56
Recipes, about, 11

S

Salads
  Classic Chicken Salad, 37
  Classic Cobb Salad, 41
  Classic Tuna Salad, 38
  Cool and Creamy Cucumber Tomato Salad, 42
  Creamy Dill and Radish "Potato" Salad, 36
  Spinach Salad with Warm Bacon Dressing, 39

Salmon
  Salmon and Egg Scramble, 19
  Salmon Croquettes, 65
Sausage
  Cheesy Sausage and Cabbage Hash, 25
  Chicken and Sausage Jambalaya, 77
  Sausage and Cheese Frittata, 14
  Zuppa Toscana (Sausage and Kale Soup), 33
Shepherd's Pie, 90–91
Shrimp and Cauliflower Grits, Coastal, 62–63
Soups, stews, and chilis
  Broccoli Cheddar Soup, 32
  Chicken and Baby Corn Chowder, 28–29
  Creamy Keto Seafood Stew, 30
  Keto Beef Chili, 35
  Southwest-Style Chicken Soup, 31
  Zuppa Toscana (Sausage and Kale Soup), 33
Spaghetti Squash, Buffalo Chicken, 68–69
Spinach
  Creamed Spinach, 57
  Spinach Salad with Warm Bacon Dressing, 39
Summer Squash Mock Apple Crumble, 108–109
Super saver recipes
  Almond Flour Crackers, 129
  Bacon-Wrapped Asparagus, 47
  Baked Egg Avocado Boats, 24
  Baked Lemon Garlic Chicken, 75
  Beef Bone Broth, 122–123
  Beef Empanadas, 87
  Breakfast Burrito Bowl, 17
  Cheese Crisps, 127

Cheesy Sausage and
Cabbage Hash, 25
Chicken Bone Broth, 124
Cinnamon Coffee
Cake, 110–111
Classic Chicken Salad, 37
Classic Chocolate
Brownies, 117
Classic Chocolate Chip
Cookies, 115
Classic Diner Hash Browns, 23
Classic Pulled Pork, 96–97
Classic Tuna Salad, 38
Coconut Chicken Adobo, 72
Creamy Dill and Radish
"Potato" Salad, 36
Crispy Chicken Tenders, 71
Crispy Pan-Roasted
Broccoli, 51
Easy Cauliflower Rice, 52
Egg Roll in a Bowl, 86
Ham and Cheese Egg Cups, 21

Keto Blueberry Pancakes, 20
Lemon Poppy Seed
Muffins, 104
Loaded Mashed
Cauliflower, 49
Magic Miracle Keto
Dough, 120–121
Panfried Tilapia, 70
Quick Pressure Cooker
Cheesecake, 105
Roasted Cabbage
Steaks, 55
Roasted Green Bean
Almandine with Blistered
Tomatoes, 48
Salmon and Egg
Scramble, 19
Salmon Croquettes, 65
Sausage and Cheese
Frittata, 14
Vegetable Broth, 125
Zucchini Noodles, 53

T
Tilapia, Panfried, 70
Tomatoes
Cool and Creamy
Cucumber Tomato
Salad, 42
Easy Guacamole, 128
Roasted Green Bean
Almandine with Blistered
Tomatoes, 48
Tuna Salad, Classic, 38
Turkey Meatballs, Sweet
and Spicy, 78–79

V
Vegetable Broth, 125

Z
Zucchini
Italian Zucchini Boats, 46
Zucchini Noodles, 53

Acknowledgments

To my husband: For his eternal patience and steadfast love over the past quarter of a century.

To my father: The best man (and cook) I know.

To my brothers: For their love, support, and great senses of humor.

To my small tribe of best friends: You know who you are, and you know you are loved.

To the low-carb and keto community: For welcoming me with open arms and open hearts, and always providing me with the inspiration and willpower to keep going.

About the Author

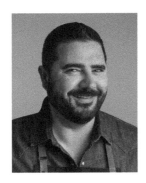

WES SHOEMAKER is the creator and personality behind the popular YouTube channel *Highfalutin' Low Carb*. Wes brings viewers into his test kitchen where, together, they search for delicious low-carb and keto recipes. His Southern style, comical flair, kitchen technique, and knowledge of keto principles have created a community of more than half a million (and growing) loyal followers who tune in to his content across YouTube, Instagram, and Facebook.

Wes is not a trained chef or nutritionist. A lover of food who was battling several nagging health issues, he created a YouTube channel in 2017 as a way to share his success with a low-carb, high-fat diet. He soon discovered that others liked to follow along on the journey, celebrating his successes and acknowledging his challenges. He turned his passion for cooking, entertaining, and content creation into a full-time job, leaving the corporate world behind.

A native Southerner, Wes currently resides in San Diego, California, with his husband of 25 years. When not behind the computer screen or in front of the camera, you can find him walking his two dogs, cooking, traveling, or gathering with small groups of friends and family.